Nature [illegible handwriting]

Voorhees

BACK TO BASICS NATURAL BEAUTY HANDBOOK

You Can Brew
Your Own Beauty
in Your Very Own Kitchen

Using only the freshest natural ingredients and the formulas in this unique and practical skin care book. For literally no more than pennies you can create cosmetics for your own personal skin type, whether dry, oily or "normal" — the right shampoos for your hair, skin cleansers and fresheners, night creams, makeup bases, soothing lotions and much, much more, all tailored to *you*! Over 200 kitchen-tested recipes that are so fresh and natural you could even eat them! And they're easy and fun to make. Plus Alexandra York's valuable professional advice on the care and feeding of a healthy and beautiful skin, a beauty course that would cost you hundreds in a spa!

BACK TO BASICS NATURAL BEAUTY HANDBOOK

HOW TO MAKE AND USE YOUR OWN NATURAL COSMETICS

ALEXANDRA YORK

 VAN NOSTRAND REINHOLD COMPANY

NEW YORK   CINCINNATI   ATLANTA   DALLAS   SAN FRANCISCO
LONDON   TORONTO   MELBOURNE

Van Nostrand Reinhold Company Regional Offices:
New York   Cincinnati   Chicago   Millbrae   Dallas

Van Nostrand Reinhold Company International Offices:
London   Toronto   Melbourne

Copyright © 1977 by Alexandra York

Library of Congress Catalog Card Number: 76-55012

ISBN: 0-442-29503-0
        0-442-29504-9 paper

All rights reserved. Certain portions of this work copyright ©1973 under title
the Natural Skin Care and Beauty Cook Book by Alexandra York. No part of
this work covered by the copyrights hereon may be reproduced or used in
any form or by any means — graphic, electronic, or mechanical, including
photocopying, recording, taping, or information storage and retrieval systems —
without written permission of the publisher.

Manufactured in the United States of America

Published by Van Nostrand Reinhold Company
450 West 33rd Street, New York, N.Y. 10001

Published simultaneously in Canada by Van Nostrand Reinhold Ltd.

15 14 13 12 11 10 9 8 7 6 5 4 3 2 1

Library of Congress Cataloging in Publication Data

York, Alexandra.
    Back to basics natural beauty handbook.

    1. Beauty, Personal.   2. Cosmetics.   I. Title.
RA778.Y55   613'.4   76-55012
ISBN 0-442-29503-0
ISBN 0-442-29504-9 pbk.

To
Every woman's man, mine included, who makes being beautiful worthwhile.

Contents

Acknowledgments

I would like to thank some very special friends for helping to test the recipes in this book: Susan Feltman, Carolyn Lane, Otto Maximilian and Georgia Tiisler. I am grateful to them all for their time, energy, inventiveness and senses of humor.

My gratitude to my personal dermatologist, Dr. Herbert Spoor, is immense. He gave me advice and answered innumerable questions over the phone as well as in person during his busy office hours. His generosity with textbooks and articles was also of much help to me.

The corner druggist, my dear Mr. Abe Davidson — former owner of Star Pharmacy — just shook his head each time I walked through the door. For his patience and invaluable help, I am more than grateful. Thanks, too, to James Viera for his information on hair.

Although I naturally engaged in lengthy and extensive research and gained a great deal from varied sources, I would like to isolate and extend my compliments and thanks to Edward Sagarin for his book *Cosmetics, Science and Technology*. I certainly stand responsible for my own interpretations and conclusions, but his concise and methodical treatment of the history of cosmetics was of special aid to me.

Thanks, too, to Jack Prather and Tommy Manno of Playboy's Resort and Country Club at Great Gorge, New Jersey, for their kind help in providing location facilities for our jacket photography so patiently done by my dear friend, Whitney Lane.

Lastly, a small nucleus of family and friends not only helped me in many specific, professional ways but supported and encouraged me personally as well. I am happy for this opportunity to thank them publicly with an enormous affection privately felt: Dr. and Mrs. Nathan Spector, Diane Creston, Erika Holzer, Barry Randell. Thank you.

A.Y.

*Beauty is worse than wine, it
intoxicates both the holder and
the beholder.*
—Johann Georg Zimmerman

Cosmetics: (1) Articles intended to be rubbed, poured, sprinkled, or sprayed on, introduced into, or otherwise applied to the human body or any part thereof for cleansing, beautifying, promoting attractiveness, or altering the appearance, and (2) Articles intended for use as a component of any such articles: except that such term shall not include soap.

—Food, Drug, and Cosmetic Act

Cosmetic (köz met'ik) *adj.* 1. beautifying or designed to beautify the complexion, hair, etc. 2. for improving the appearance by the removal or correction of blemishes or deformities, esp. of the face — *n.* any cosmetic preparation for application to the skin, hair, etc. as rouge and powder.

—Webster's New World Dictionary

Introduction

Most actresses who are in the business of beauty are rich, successful, established women. They sell their own lines of cosmetics and I think it's wonderful.

When I first became interested in "Back to Basics" cosmetics several years ago, I was a relatively new and unknown actress who couldn't afford to buy the pots of beauty the other actresses sold, let alone start my own line.

And that's how *I* got into the beauty business. I began making my own concoctions out of necessity. Beauty is an important aspect of every actress's life, and I needed to find a way to save my face while I saved my money.

After brewing my own cosmetics for a considerable time now, I find to my delight that:

1. it is fascinating and fun;
2. it works;
3. it costs pennies to do. . .I should be rich by now with the money I've saved. (The most expensive cream in the book costs about seventy-five cents to make);
4. cosmetics, at last, are removed from the realm of the unknown. I know *what's* in my creams, *how much* is in there and best of all *why* it's in there;
5. every beauty aid I use is custom created for my very own skin. And I couldn't touch the cost, freshness or quality with a "store bought" product.

The only possible drawback I've been able to discover is that I occasionally eat my ingredients by mistake.

I had been sharing my recipes with friends since I conjured up my first batch and suddenly realized that if we were so excited over the results, there must be many other women in the country who would enjoy brewing their own beauty, too.

And that's when I decided to compile this "do it yourself" skin care manual.

Cosmetics themselves are one of the means by which we achieve or preserve a healthy, beautiful skin. But in order for the means to be *meaningful*, they have to fulfill the requirements of that skin; and in order to know what the requirements of the skin are, we must investigate and understand the nature of the skin itself.

This understanding is necessary whether one elects to make products at home or to buy them in the store — if one wants to do either intelligently.

So in response to and respect for my readers who demand to know the "whys" and "wherefores" of skin care, I have attempted to illuminate the principles behind the products as well as offer at-home recipes on how to make them.

I hope you'll have as much fun in the exploration of the subject and the conjuring-up of the cosmetics as I have had, and I am confident that you will be delighted with the results.

One word of advice: if one day you find my line of cosmetics on the shelf. . .just remember. . .I'll have used the recipes from this book.

BACK TO BASICS
NATURAL
BEAUTY
HANDBOOK

1

A Good Birthday Suit
Is Never Out of Style

Beauty is the virtue of the body as virtue is the beauty of the soul.
—Ralph Waldo Emerson

Most of us don't think of the skin as an organ. But it is, and it's the largest organ of our entire body. The surface covers about nineteen square feet, weighs an average of seven pounds, and varies in thickness from one-thirty second to one-eighth of an inch. This organ, which is 98 percent protein, is not only large but complex as well. *One square inch* of skin contains approximately three yards of blood vessels, three hundred sweat glands, twelve yards of nerves, six hundred nerve endings, thirty hairs, and forty-five oil glands!

When you view the subject of health and beauty with these statistics in mind, you begin to understand that it's not just vanity but good common sense to care for this precious protective covering.

A healthy, hence beautiful, skin is soft to the touch, yet firm, because of an inherent elasticity. It is moist, with a definite acid balance. In texture, good skin is smooth and fine-grained. In color, it is uniform and glows. . .with life.

Unfortunately, most of the skin's basic attributes — color, texture, aging tendencies — are inherited. Fortunately, we live in the age of science where specialists can tell us what to do with our inherited package to correct Nature's mistakes.

The trick lies in the examination and evaluation of science's vital information in order to apply it to our own individual skins. In order to perform that little gymnastic, it's necessary to understand something about this marvelous organ. It's true that all skins are individual in some respects, but it's also true that all skins are alike in some respects.

Everyone's skin, for example, is made up of two main layers. The outermost layer, the one that protects everything underneath, is called the *epidermis.* Beside its main occupation as "protector" of all the other organs, it also contains a rich nerve supply. This nerve network responds to touch, pain, and pressure, as well as to heat and cold. . . sending sensory messages to the brain and acting as a thermostat reporting the temperature outside so that the system can adjust its heaters and air conditioners inside to keep you comfortable.

The epidermis itself has several layers, but it's necessary here to examine only the bottom layer — technically termed the *basal layer.* It is the function of the cells of this layer to continually renew the life of your skin. They divide, and while the newly created cells carry on the life processes the original cells are carried progressively to the surface of the skin. Because they cannot survive exposure to air and water, they grow old there and eventually die. Then they are gradually shed. It's because of this very efficient system of sloughing off the old, dead skin only to reveal new, fresh skin that we are able to maintain a soft, young-looking skin. A not unimportant side benefit of this process is the skin's built-in ability to eradicate superficial scars in this manner.

Immediately beneath the epidermis — which literally means "upon the dermis" — is situated, logically enough. . . the *dermis.* This second layer is sometimes referred to as the "true skin." It's made up of a protein fiber which accounts for most of the skin's elasticity. Time alone weakens the fiber and so, with age, the elasticity is diminished, the skin

CROSS SECTION OF SKIN

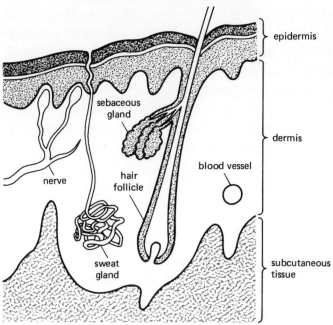

becomes looser and thinner, and wrinkles begin to appear.

The dermis extends deeper into kind of a cushion of fatty subcutaneous tissue, tissue with the gift of life, for it has the very special function of feeding the skin and rendering it free from toxins and waste materials. And that's only on the inside!

There are also what we might think of as inside-outside workers such as the sebaceous or oil glands. At the base of every hair on your body is a private little oil well. These bottomless wells provide a protective oil balance called *sebum* which appears on the surface of the skin. I'm sure you've been aware of visible oil on your own or someone else's forehead. It's most apparent there because the center of the forehead, along with the scalp, nose, and chin, contain more sebaceous glands than any other area of the entire body. If you blot the oil off, it will replace itself within a short time. This is simply your oil glands striving to protect you. Nobody told them we find it undesirable beautywise, so every time we get rid of excess oil on the surface they send up more to take its place. And they do it all over the body.

Many women have complexion problems around menstruation time. That's because there's a rise in the activity of the sebaceous glands on about the twelfth or fifteenth day of the menstrual cycle and then this rather high level is maintained until the onset of menstruation. So if you experience breakouts on your face each month, your oil wells may be to blame.

The entire skin organ has as its special duty the eliminative functions of the body. It virtually *breathes* for the body through the pores in very much the same manner as the lungs, but of course on a much smaller scale. Oxygen is taken in and carbon dioxide is discharged. Water, too, is eliminated — approximately a pint of it on an average day. (Now you see the need for moisturizing creams.) The skin also rids the body of any toxins that may be harmful.

I've already mentioned the oils that come to the surface for elimination by the skin. Well, some of them don't always make it and become trapped. If they can't be secreted, the skin then has the ability to oxidize them. This *forces* them out. In the form of a blemish.

Besides the capacity to eliminate substances from the system, the skin is also able to do the reverse. It has a limited ability to absorb. "Limited" because if it could take things in as readily as it lets them out we'd all be dead. It seems to have the very good discriminative ability to absorb (predominately via the hair follicles and sebaceous glands) those things that help the body — like natural oils from a good cream — and at the same time refuse admission to poisons and toxins in the air.

Aside from exotic trappings like oil wells and convenient powers of eliminating unwanted visitors, the skin also possesses permanent inhabitants — the "flora" family.

Flora is the term used to designate the many types of bacteria that make the skin their home. Don't let it concern you. There are desirable members of the flora family as well as undesirable ones, just as in any family. The bacteria differ from one individual to the next, from one region of the body to another, as well as from day to day and month to month in the same body. Their favorite places to live are the very openings through which the oil wells send their precious cargo, and if the bacteria living there at the time aren't the desirable ones a pimple is on its way. This is one of the innumerable reasons the skin must be kept immaculately clean.

One of the precautions the skin takes to keep out harmful bacteria and other infection is to cloak itself with an *acid mantle*. It's actually a matter of maintaining the proper acid-alkaline balance, but for good health the balance must lean toward the acid, so it has been termed an acid mantle. This is what the *pH factor* you may have heard of is all about. pH is a method of measuring the acidity or alkalinity of any substance you wish to test.

You can buy nitrazine paper at the drugstore. It's yellow and comes in a little dispenser. When you dip it into your cosmetic, bath oil, soap, etc., it turns color. There's a color scale right on the package ranging from pH 4.5 to pH 7.5. Anything that registers 7 or below is acidic. Anything that registers above 7 is alkaline.

The acid mantle or balance of the skin hovers between 4.2 and 5.6, so of course the best products to use on your face would be those which fall within that range. Anything above a pH 7 level, if used at all, should be followed by a skin freshener to restore the skin's normal acidity for the sake of its health.

Washing your face with soap and water will be examined later, but it's appropriate to note here that, while I have tested dozens of soaps with nitrazine paper, I have found only a few with the same acidity level as the skin.

The skin ages soon enough all by itself without any additional assistance from cleansers and beauty aids that "aid" you only to premature lines and wrinkles.

While touching on that subject, I have heartening news for women with oily skin. After about the age of thirty, the skin just naturally becomes drier. This is the age when most women will begin to see lines near the eyes and mouth.   But not you (now lucky) ladies with the same oily skin that plagued you from adolescence till now. Since your sebaceous glands are naturally overactive, they'll keep you in soft, dewy skin years longer than your dry-skinned sisters who now need to stimulate and replenish their own oil wells with primers from a bottle.

Beautiful skin, no matter what the type, however, demands constant care to resist the aging process.   And the earlier you start, the better.   You'll notice the loss of elasticity first in your neck. This is a warning signal, and the face is next.   Massaging properly with moisturizing creams will help tone the underlying muscles of the face and slow down the inevitable.   And that's precisely what we're attempting to accomplish with all skins.   You can't *stop* the process of aging, but you surely can slow it down.   And the way to do that is to maintain a healthy skin that is cleansed, toned, moisturized, and cared for every day of your life.

Caring for the skin externally is not, of course, *everything* that the skin requires to stay young and beautiful.

What goes *onto* your body surely is important — this entire book is dedicated to that aspect of beauty alone — but never underestimate the value of what goes *into* your body as well.

A nutritious, balanced diet is crucial. Lots of protein — lean meats, fish, poultry, and eggs — plus fruits, vegetables, dairy products, and adequate quantities of water all help to keep you strong, healthy, and functioning efficiently on the inside.   If your internal organs are malfunctioning, the resulting toxins can spread to the bloodstream where they will be transported to the skin for elimination. This procedure is normal and proper, but the frequency of such a demand on the skin is a factor determining its own health. It's possible to literally overwork the skin organ. Elasticity, texture, and color can all be adversely affected.

If the *what* goes into your body is critical, the *how much* is important, too. If the proportion is not sufficient, it could result in a vitamin deficiency. There is rather impressive evidence that lack of vitamins — especially A (green and yellow vegetables), D (milk), and B (liver) — directly affect the health of the skin. These can be supplemented with foods such as cod liver oil (vitamins A and D) and brewer's yeast (vitamin B) or with vitamin pills, but every effort should be made to assure the skin the benefit of these vitamins. If vitamin C (the infection-fighting vitamin) is insufficient in the diet, the skin may also mirror the loss.

My purpose here is not to offer a dissertation on nutrition, but merely to spotlight the subject of diet in general for your further inquiry.

A parallel consideration which also has an effect for good or ill on the skin is *exercise*. The fitness of the rest of your body is reflected in the appearance of your skin. Exercise stimulates all internal organs to function smoothly, it distributes the nutrients just discussed, it tones the muscles, and it eradicates fatigue and stress. It gets that wonderful machine which is your body *moving*. It encourages *life*.

It's necessary to attend to your whole package, not just the wrapping. Care for the health of your whole body. . . outside *and* inside. Your *skin*, and its resulting health and beauty, will merely declare to the world the well-being of the body it surrounds.

HOW TO FIND YOUR OWN SKIN TYPE

Before you learn how to care for your skin, you must learn just what type of skin you have. Cosmeticians divide these types into three categories: normal, oily, and dry. It's also possible to have a combination of any of these three groups on the same face. For example, you might have an oily "T" zone (forehead, nose, and chin) with the rest of the face skin dry. Any combination you may have is aptly labeled a *combination* skin. It's a bit of trouble, practically speaking, because you have to care for each zone individually, so it's necessary to use a few more beauty aids. The great majority of women *do* have combination skins, however, so this is just another excellent reason to save money on cosmetics by making your own.

Even if you elect to buy cleansers and creams, you can't possibly do it intelligently without knowing your skin type. And if you decide to make your own, you need to know your type in order to select recipes. Thorough familiarity with your skin type is also necessary in order to purchase makeup. For example, if you find you possess a dry skin, you'll want to make sure to buy oil-based foundations and liquid or cream blushers. If you have oily skin, you'll require oil-absorbing makeup and dry cheek colors.

The simplest way to find your skin type (and also the most enjoyable) is to go to a salon and have an analysis and a facial. It's a delicious treat and can prove to be continually beneficial even after you start your at-home routine. Most salons suggest that you come once a month for a professional facial and then maintain a regular beauty program at home between visits. At the salon, they'll settle you into a reclining lounge, tuck you in with a pretty coverlet, and then proceed to cleanse and pamper your face, neck, and shoulders for an hour or more. Cleopatra herself never had it so good. Most salons will try to sell you their products after the facial, so forewarned is forearmed. Just tell them firmly that you love their facials but you have your own custom line of cosmetics and are very happy with them. (As I know you will be.)

You don't *need* a professional analysis, however. So if there's no salon in your town, or if you don't want to spend the money (they're expensive), or if you're just not interested in that sort of thing, you can very easily analyze your own skin. Once you know your skin type, it's merely a matter of selecting recipes and opening the jar to a whole new way of life for your face.

First, get hold of a magnifying mirror if you can. It's not absolutely necessary, so don't run out and buy one. But if you have one handy it will make the job easier. Now look carefully (and honestly) at your face. The following guide will help you make a correct analysis.

NORMAL SKIN

This is the most rare type of all, so I can't imagine why it's called *normal* skin. It's the kind of skin we're all trying to achieve. If you find it's your type, consider yourself chosen and be certain to *take care of it* to keep it that way. Normal skin is young, fresh, firm, moist, finegrained, supple skin with a smooth texture. It is free from blemishes.

You must keep an eye on this type of skin because, as I mentioned earlier in this chapter, around the age of thirty, skin by its very nature begins to get drier. Eventually, as you get older, you will have dry skin, so watch for it carefully and when it arrives switch to a dry skin care routine. The first signs will be a taut feeling to your face when the weather turns cold and a general sensitivity to the elements. Also, if you wash with most soaps (which will probably speed you toward those "dry" days), you'll experience a tight feeling afterward.

DRY OR DEHYDRATED SKIN

If you have dry skin, it's a sign of sluggish or underactive oil glands and/or the inability of your skin to produce or retain enough water moisture. It will have a tendency toward early lines and wrinkles, so if you're under thirty and are starting to discover small lines in the eye or mouth area already you've probably got dry skin.

Other clues to this skin type are the presence of small pore openings and fine lines on a thin skin. With your fingertips, push the skin upward. If you see tiny little lines form, that's a pretty sure sign. If you burn or peel easily in the sun and chap easily in the wind and cold, and if you get a "tight" feeling in cold weather or after a soap and water wash, you can be assured of your diagnosis. If your skin occasionally appears or feels parched and has a tendency to flake, turn immediately to the recipe section. There's not a moment to lose.

Dry skin needs not only constant vigil but also protection against the elements. You'll need the benefits of a moisturizing cream at all times but especially in winter when the artificial heat in your house results in a loss of humidity in the air, hence a loss of moisture in your skin.

A deep tan is not for you, whether from the beach or the ski slopes. Be sure to always smooth on a good sunscreen with an oil base. Your skin can be positively stunning because it is so delicate, but you have to pamper it as you would any fragile flower.

OILY SKIN

If you were the dismayed owner of an acne condition during adolescence you probably still have oily skin now. Not always, of course, because nerves, diet, hormonal imbalance, and innumerable other factors play a significant role in creating skin problems. So look for other signs to support your suspicion. If your skin has a glossy (I won't say "greasy" but take a look for it anyway) appearance, it may be the surface evidence of an oily condition. If your skin is susceptible to blackheads and/or small bumps beneath the surface, you are likely to fall into this skin category. Enlarged pores are another phenomenon to check for.

If you decide your skin is oily and you're under thirty, it's a type to be relentlessly cared for. And not with tender, loving care, but with firm, no-nonsense discipline. If you're over thirty, your skin will continue getting lovelier each year as your extra oil output moistens it to a beautiful "normal" condition. Watch for indications that your overactive oil wells are slowing down and switch recipes accordingly.

When you apply cosmetics on this skin type, you must exercise caution in one respect. Caring for an oily skin does not mean robbing it of *all* of its oils. If you strip away all of these natural moisturizers, your skin will not be able to maintain the necessary balance of oils and water that it properly needs. What you must do is keep the face free of *excess* oiliness. That's the reason why I include ingredients in the Protection creams (which are specifically designed for oily skins) which will help your skin retain its natural oils and water without adding more. If you kept your skin absolutely dry of oils, you'd soon experience the same early aging tendencies as a person with dry skin.

COMBINATION SKIN

The most frequent combination of *combination* skin is part oily and part normal or dry. You can readily see the excess oil on the forehead and possibly the nose area. Perhaps it's not so discernible on the chin, but if you have a blemish problem (however sporadic) in that zone, the chin is probably oily, too. Check for enlarged pores and tiny black- or whiteheads hiding under the surface of the skin which give it a "grainy" appearance. The cheeks, including the jaw line and the outer edges of the forehead will most likely be dry or normal. Scrutinize all sections of your face carefully to determine the type of each.

Combination skin requires slightly more effort than the other types, but it's not formidable. You must simply treat and care for each zone separately. Oily lotions and masks for the areas needing them and dry or normal treatments for the rest. Once you get into the swing of a routine with the appropriate products, you'll be able to juggle the different bottles deftly. Also, if it gives you any comfort, most women fall into this category.

TROUBLED SKIN

This isn't technically a skin *type* but a skin *condition.* And you won't have any difficulty spotting it. It can be caused by so many things — poor diet, hormonal changes, nerves, improper skin hygiene — that you must plan on taking care of it in a very special way. And on a long-term basis. You'll find specific information and programs to follow in Chapter Six which is devoted to the subject.

ALL TYPES

Each skin type demands a routine specifically designed to meet its individual needs. Guidelines for this purpose are outlined in Chapter Five, but the general program is the same. All types require thorough cleansing and care. In the morning and certainly again before retiring, you will want to use a deep cream cleansing to unclog the pores of dirt and grime and let the skin breathe in order to fulfill its role as an eliminative organ. If you wish to use a soap and water wash, it would come next. The all-important skin freshener follows to restore the pH factor (should it be necessary), tone and freshen the skin, as well as finish the cleaning job. Next comes eye cream to soften and diminish the appearance of wrinkles around the eye area. Lastly, the application of a moisturizing or protection cream, which will soften and lubricate the skin as well as help it to maintain its vital oil and water balance. This cream, in addition, protects the skin under makeup and against the elements.

You may ask "is that all?" — and understandably so. With all of the specialty products on the market, it would surely be reasonable to wonder about the possible added value of ultrarich night creams, under-makeup moisturizers, etc.

In my judgment, any more than the previously itemized beauty aids is superfluous for daily skin care. *All* of the recipes in this book produce ultrarich creams. And a good cream moisturizes, softens, and protects your skin at any hour. . . be it day or night.

I can find no valid reason to have separate beauty aids for morning, for under makeup, and for before bed except possibly the fun of variety. If this appeals to you, then by all means prepare as many concoctions as you like and enjoy them at any time you like. The only point I want to communicate is that the *result* will be the same as if you'd used the same product for each purpose.

The program still goes as follows: 1) cleanse with a cream; 2) an optional soap and water wash; 3) further cleanse, freshen, and tone with a skin freshener; 4) moisturize and protect with a second cream. Voila and fini!

The procedure is essentially the same for all skins. However, the *products used* are drastically different since each skin type needs help in its own special way.

Examine your skin carefully from time to time to reaffirm your type. If it has changed, you'll get to know another recipe section as you meet your skin's new requirements.

2

The Care and Feeding of Your Face

Personal beauty is a greater recommendation than any letter of introduction.

—*Aristotle*

Your face is the only part of your body where all of your beauty is visible at one time. A healthy physical beauty appears in the texture and color of your skin, and this in turn becomes the setting for your eyes which express a healthy mental beauty. The combination can be something to behold.

Unfortunately, the skin of the face is the most exposed to weather, gets the least exercise, and ages first. Because of these facts, it's natural *and proper* for every woman to give it a reasonable amount of consideration and attention.

The *first* consideration, however, goes not to your skin but to a room. The one sometimes referred to as your kitchen. When you're out there brewing a batch of beauty in your pots, that room can no longer be labeled a mere "kitchen." It must then become a beauty brewery of the first order, so before you start flexing your creative muscles. . .get prepared.

You don't have to keep separate utensils for making your beauty aids (if you keep them immaculately clean) because you'll be using natural ingredients. I keep all of my beauty tools special because it's more dramatic. (And also, I can be sure that any leftover beeswax won't end up in my mint peas for dinner.) But it certainly isn't necessary, so there's no need to purchase a brand new set of cookware.

Old or new, here's a list of what you'll need:

1 fair-size sauce pan 1 medium sauce pan 1 small sauce pan	At the dimestore, I got three stainless steel sauce pans that nest together. They're perfect in size: the largest for waxes and mixing, the medium for oils, and the smallest for waters when you're brewing creams.
1 very small sauce pan	I use one of those pretty copper butter warmers. It can be really small because you'll only use it to premelt oils that come in solid form (like cocoa butter) before adding them to the other liquid oils.
1 wire whisk *or* egg beater *or* electric beater	I use the wire whisk because I want to look like a French chef in case any photographer from *Vogue* is secretly taking pictures from a neighboring building, but the electric beater is by far the fastest and most efficient.
1 or 2 sets measuring spoons	
1 measuring cup	
1 one-ounce shot glass	This becomes a handy little measuring cup. I have indicated many measurements in ounces. You can use a measuring cup, but the shot glass is faster and can even add to the atmosphere. Check to see if yours holds exactly 1 ounce (that's 2 tablespoons).

1 small funnel

1 small strainer
   (fine)

1 colander   There is really no need for this except
                    that I have all of my things hanging
                    from a rack on the ceiling and it looks
                    very happy up there — it's yellow — so
                    I use it for draining fruits and vege-
                    tables for the recipes.

1 blender   You can make all of the recipes with-
                    out one by mashing and straining,
                    but I'd give up everything else in the
                    brewery *and* the kitchen before I'd
                    give up that blender. (If you're in the
                    market for a blender, be sure to get
                    one that does not require liquid in
                    order to blend).

1 juicer   Again, you don't *need* this; it just
                    makes it easier.

As I mentioned previously, you may or may not elect
to keep your beauty *utensils* separate and together. However, I would strongly suggest that you do keep your
ingredients separate and apart from your other food-
stuffs; otherwise you'll eat them by mistake, and there
goes your beauty. . .right down the gullet.

In one cupboard keep a box — I have a topless shoe box
covered with pretty paper — for your store of cocoa butter,
beeswax, lanolin, etc.; things that don't need refrigeration.

Then, in the refrigerator, set aside one crisper for
beauty fruits and vegetables. You can do this one of
two ways. Either buy foods especially for the beauty

recipes (cucumbers, strawberries, lemons, etc.), keep them there until you use them, and then feed your family the leftovers. . .or, when you have leftovers from your meals that could be used in the beauty concoctions, put them in the crisper and select recipes to match.

One other thing. Save a little space next to your beauty box in the cupboard — or add another box — for a collection of pretty bottles and jars. You'll probably find as you get more and more involved and interested in homemade cosmetics that when you buy food for *eating* purposes you'll be sold by a container that can later be used to hold your beauty elixirs.

Now you have a beauty cookery. Time to talk about cooking.

THE INGREDIENTS

Before you start on any of these recipes, of course, you'll need to purchase the ingredients. You'll find why each one is used and where to buy it in Chapter Eleven, The Beauty Gourmet's Glossary. You'll also find there a list of measurements to help you cut or double recipes should you desire to do so.

When you purchase your "stuff," there are a few points to remember. Products from the drugstore won't spoil, so buy them in large quantities. Many of the same ingredients can be used in several different recipes, and you'll save money buying in bulk. (*Talk* to your druggist about this. Let him know you'd like to save 10 or 20 percent and find out what he can do for you. Make *friends* with your druggist!) If you don't want a large supply yourself, divvy it up among your friends and divide the cost.

When buying rose water, try to get "double strength" rose water and then dilute it — half rose water to half plain water — at home.

As you probably are already aware, natural oils become rancid if left in a cupboard, so once they're opened, keep them in the refrigerator.

The purposes of the creams — cleansing, moisturizing, protecting — vary. And since the purpose dictates the ingredients used, ingredients also vary. But the rationale behind the choice of basic ingredients and the principles of making the creams themselves apply to any type of cream.

Creams are basically a mixture of oils, waxes, and water with a little emulsifier to hold them together. This means any creams. . .whether you buy them or make them. It's the *choice* and *quality* of the oils, waxes, and waters that will make your homemade creams far superior to most any you could buy.

To get you acquainted with some of the reasons for the ingredients you'll be using, I'll explore some of the more interesting ones here. For a more complete description, consult Chapter Eleven.

You're going to use honey beeswax, which is a substance secreted by and found in the honeycombs of bees. It's a natural product that will not clog pores like paraffin may which is used in many commercial products. Beeswax also acts as a skin softener.

Spermaceti is another natural skin-softening wax that comes from the head of a whale. Since it is rather difficult to obtain it from the original source, your druggist will oblige you.

You can use plain or distilled water in any of these recipes, but I prefer some of the more refreshing liquids like witch hazel which is cooling, rose water or extracts which offer delightful aromas, or fresh fruit juices which have both attributes. Fruit juices also have beneficial astringent qualities.

The most important ingredients of all are the *oils*. Some oils are able to penetrate — or be absorbed by — the skin. Some oils are not.

Normal and dry skins can most definitely benefit from a penetrating oil. If the sebaceous glands are sluggish and not capable of putting out enough oil of their own to lubricate and soften the skin, the oils absorbed from a good cream can stimulate the glands to secrete more oil themselves and at the same time supplement the supply.

In the instance of oily skin, absorbing *more* oil into already overactive sebaceous glands would only amplify the problem. A *non-penetrable* cream, on the other hand, will lubricate and soften the *surface* of the skin and perform its primary service of helping the skin retain *water* without adding more *oil* to the system.

Natural animal or vegetable oils have the power to penetrate the skin. Mineral oils do not. Therefore, recipes in this book are specifically geared to the individual needs of individual skin types.

Mineral oils are used as a base for cleansing and "protection" creams for *oily skins.*

Liquid vegetable oils are used as a base for cleansing and "moisturizing" creams for *normal and dry skins.* If you're wondering why I specify *liquid* vegetable oils over solids or animal fats, it's because liquid fats penetrate better and faster than solid ones. Luckily, then, I was able to eliminate the use of lard, suet, and goose grease at the outset. That left vegetable and animal fats in liquid form. Since vegetable oils are plentiful, relatively inexpensive, with great varieties in kind — and animal oils are virtually nonexistent on the market — I have conveniently decided to use vegetable oils.

Of the vegetable oils, almond oil is believed to be the best (it's also the most expensive), with virgin olive oil running a close second (it's the second most expensive... you figure it out: are they good because they're expensive or expensive because they're good?). Others which are excellent (much less expensive and perhaps just as good) are any other natural vegetable oils you would like to buy. This includes coconut, cottonseed, peanut, corn, peach or apricot kernel, sesame, safflower, soy, avocado. . . a practically limitless list. In all of the cream recipes for normal or dry skin, feel free to substitute and use whatever vegetable oil you happen to have in the house.

Almost every type of cream for *any* type skin that is *commercially* available is made with a mineral oil base. For two valid reasons. One, it is the cheapest oil you can buy. And two, it has an unlimited shelf life as opposed to vegetable oil-based creams which tend to become rancid rather quickly and require more substantive preservatives.

For oily skins, these mineral oil-based creams, should you decide to purchase them, would not only be fine but advisable.

In recent years, the trend has been toward natural, *vegetable oil*-based creams. They are usually more expensive *and*, like the mineral oil-based creams, they are *not suitable* for all types of skins   Only *normal* and *dry skins*, will benefit from these moisturizers.

In any case, the ingredients are not usually listed on the package in any language remotely understandable to the layman. Because of this, you might buy an "almond" moisturizing cream assuming (without any evidence) that the cream is made with almond oil. It may have one drop of almond oil and the rest mineral oil for all you know. Or it may only have an almond *scent* and no vegetable oil at all. This is true of any commercial cosmetic, whether you purchase it at a drug, department, or health food store.

The same uncertainty surrounds the current flood of "fruit" and "vegetable" creams. If you read carefully, you'll find that most of the cosmetics labeled "cucumber" or "lemon" or "strawberry," etc., do not say the creams are *made* with cucumbers, lemons, strawberries, etc. They talk about the fresh *smell* which would indicate that fruit or vegetable *aromas* have been added to a cream made of. . .what?   Sometimes they specify "extract," which is better, but you still don't know whether it's natural or synthetic or how much of it is actually in the cream.

I would like to stress that, in my judgment, none of these practices on the part of the cosmetic industry is illegal or even immoral.   If you wish to buy their products, that is surely your prerogative.   There is room in the beauty world for both "store bought" and homemade cosmetics.   We can be grateful that we have such a limitless choice.

But I would like to encourage you to wonder a bit about what you're actually getting, or may be getting, when you buy.   If you make your own cosmetics, you know.

This, of course, is one of the major advantages of homemade beauty aids.   You know exactly *what* is in them, *how much* of it is in them, and, after reading this book, *why* it is in them.   As a result, you can select and tailor recipes to fulfill your very own, individual preferences and requirements.   You are also assured of the purity and freshness of the ingredients.   In other words, *you* are in direct control of which substances come into contact with your skin.

Allergy control is another excellent reason for making cosmetics at home.   If you make the product yourself, and you do experience a reaction, you can substitute one ingredient at a time, discover which one is the culprit, and eliminate it from any future products.   If you *buy* a cosmetic and find you are sensitive to it, it's impossible to know specifically which substance is triggering the reaction.   You can spend a lot of money hopping from one brand to another, armed only with the hope that the next one won't contain "whatever it was" that is spelling trouble for you.

Technically, you should apply the "patch test" with any product — store bought or homemade — that is going to be used on your body. Even hypoallergenic, dermatologist-tested, natural, organic cosmetics could be incompatible with your skin. It's not probable but always possible to experience an allergic reaction to a substance at any given time even if you have never previously experienced such a reaction. So do the "patch test" just as a safeguard. Rub a small amount of any cream, lotion, or makeup on the inside of your elbow. Cover it lightly with a bandage and leave it for twenty-four hours. If any redness or rash occurs, don't use the product.

The issue of vitamins applied in cream or oil form to the skin should be examined here because you will find recipes that include vitamin ingredients.

It is true that the skin benefits from vitamins, especially A, D, and B when taken into the body via food (or supplements). They perform an important role in building and maintaining the tissues and cell structure of the skin.

It is also true that vitamins rubbed topically on the surface of the skin have been detected *within* the system of a body previously deficient in the vitamin in question. However, the vitamins so applied have been detected in *minute* quantities only.

It's only logical. If you stop to consider the small amount of actual vitamin in a jar of cream and then think of the little dab of the cream that goes on your face, the whole subject becomes rather farfetched.

Even if you applied the vitamin full strength — using the entire contents of a vitamin capsule, for example — there is not sufficient proof that it is effective from the outside-*in*. Once it reaches the internal system, it may be beneficial from the inside-*out* as previously mentioned; but even then it would be more direct to pop the pill in your mouth instead of rubbing it on your face.

There are some startling "stories" about spectacular success achieved by applying vitamin oils externally, but the tests were not, to my mind, scientific enough to *prove* anything.

To conclude: If you are still interested in checking the subject out for yourself, vitamin recipes are included throughout the book. (I have not included vitamins, however, in face creams for oily skins. There is some evidence that the presence of vitamins A and D causes mineral oil to penetrate the skin. This would not be good for oily skins. So to stay on the safe side, I have elected to omit vitamin creams for this skin type.)

My reasons for offering any of them to you even when I, personally, don't believe in them are as follows: 1) apparently the application of vitamins to the surface of the skin does no harm; 2) the creams, masks, lotions, etc., in which vitamin ingredients appear are rich and beneficial *without* the addition of the vitamins, so I know you will still get the skin care you need; 3) if you make vitamin products at *home*, at least you'll be investing nickels and dimes rather than dollars into a beauty aid that may or may not "work"; 4) if you're able to make it and try it, it gives you the opportunity to "see for yourself."

Whether you decide to put vitamin pills on your face or in it, read on and learn how to make some of these luscious creams I've been promising you.

PROCEDURES AND TIPS FOR MAKING CREAMS

The making of creams is really very simple. You know now that they are basically a combination of waxes, oils, and waters. As a general rule for preparation, just remember that the waxes are melted together first (over *LOW* heat), the oils warmed and beaten into the waxes, and the heated waters dribbled slowly and beaten into that mixture. And that's all there is to it. Once you've got the ingredients together, it will take approximately 5 to 15 minutes from start to finish.

The creams will vary in consistency. It's really a matter of personal preference whether you want a soft or firm cream; the important factor is what's *in* the cream. Sometimes the consistency will firm slightly after the cream sits for a few hours. If this happens, simply rewhip the cream lightly with a fork and it will then remain soft and fluffy.

And, dear reader, these creams are ultrarich. *Use only a little.* (If you find you're using more than one ounce of cream every couple of months, you're probably using too much.) If you have normal or dry skin, give the cream a few moments to penetrate. Then blot any excess off your face with a tissue.

After you make one of these creams for the first time, if you'd like to change its texture you can. Simply add more beeswax if you want it firmer, more oil if you want it softer. If you wish to change the scent, use any flavor extract in place of whatever water is called for, *or* substitute a scented oil for part of the vegetable or mineral oil called for in the recipe. (When heating extracts, use a low heat. A high flame can create a "flaming" extract.)

If waxes harden on spoons or in pots, heat the utensil over boiling water and, when the wax is melted again, wash quickly with hot, soapy water and a steel wool pad. (The way to avoid this is to wash pots and spoons by the same method immediately after using them.)

Because beeswax, and sometimes spermaceti, usually come in cake form, it's more convenient to melt it down and measure it out in advance than to melt and measure for each individual recipe.

Cut some aluminum foil into four- to six-inch squares. Form a little cup out of each square and set the little cups out on the cabinet in a row. Next, melt a cake or two of beeswax (over *LOW* heat) and measure 1 teaspoon of the liquid wax into each cup. When the wax hardens, wrap the rest of the cup around the "whole ball of wax" and pop the foil into a box. If a recipe calls for 2 tea-spoons of wax, unwrap two balls and melt them down again. If it calls for 1 tablespoon, unwrap three balls, and so on. If you get your friends in on this, you can trade six balls of beeswax for six balls of spermaceti (or more, depending on your business acumen and nerve).

Another method for measuring solid waxes or fats — such as cocoa butter or coconut oil — is to utilize water, a measuring cup, and the principle of displacement. Example: if the recipe calls for 1 ounce of cocoa butter, fill a measuring cup with 1 ounce of water. Drop some cocoa butter into the water and keep adding more of it, a little at a time, until the water level reaches 2 ounces. Then pour out the water. The remaining cocoa butter will measure 1 ounce when melted down.

As for the color of some of the creams, don't be surprised. The first cream I ever made was a beautiful mint-green, and then as I stood there gloating it turned a kind of sick gray-green right before my very eyes. I learned soon enough that it's not the appearance of the cream (most of them are naturally pretty) but how it works that is all-important. (If you use stainless steel rather than alumi-num pots the creams will come out a nicer color.) The beautiful *color* of a cream, however, is not what pro-motes a beautiful *skin*. These cosmetics have no preserva-tives, permanent emulsifiers, synthetics, or added coloring like the ones you buy. Consequently, they don't come every color of the rainbow. I think you'll quickly dis-cover, however, that their pot of gold is lovelier, and when you begin to see the results you won't care what color they are. If it really matters to you, just add a drop or two of any natural food coloring you desire. . .then you can have all the baby pinks, greens and yellows you wish.

You'll notice that whenever perishable ingredients are included in the recipe, I specify refrigeration. It is true that if you cool them, they will last longer. I, however, do not keep mine in the fridge and most of them last for months, certainly long enough to use them up. Be sure your hands are clean before dipping fingers into anything that goes on your face to avoid adding unwanted bacteria.

Now recipes. Get started and have some fun making your own pots of gold, or green, or gray and refrigerate them or not. But I guarantee the first recipe to last indefinitely and be white as Crisco.

CLEANSING CREAMS

The first purpose of a cleansing cream is to remove make-up, surface grime, and accumulated oils from the face and throat. That gets you clean on the outside. You get an internal cleaning too. As you gently massage the cream onto your face, the circulation of the blood is increased, bringing oxygen to the surface to feed the skin. Then, on its return trip, the blood takes along with it any waste products that may be hiding near the surface. If, before you remove the cream, you gently scrub the

APPLYING CLEANSING CREAM

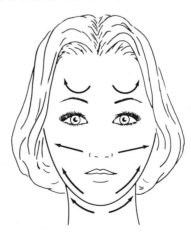

face with a natural bristle complexion brush, you can effectively remove dead skin cells that have accumulated on the surface waiting to be sloughed off. Whether you decide to use your fingers or a brush, remove the cream with several clean tissues or a warm, wet washcloth. (If you wear makeup, I recommend the tissues because makeup does not always wash out of the cloths).

Oily skins: If you're discriminating in your selection, you can benefit from the drying effect of a soap and water wash *following* the cleansing cream.

As far as normal and dry skins are concerned, there seems to be a never-ending controversy among skin authorities concerning the use of soap as a facial cleanser. Some recommend its use as long as it contains a germicide. Others say to use soap as long as it *doesn't* contain a germicide. Health food advocates suggest the use of soap as long as it is made of natural ingredients — like cucumbers, oatmeal, etc. Still others, concerned with the acid-alkaline balance, suggest any soap rendering the same pH factor as the skin. (Very few, by the way; I've tested them.)

USING COMPLEXION BRUSH

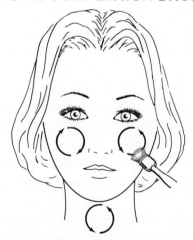

TISSUING OFF CLEANSING CREAM

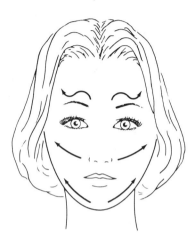

What to do with all of this contradictory information? My advice is to use a cleansing cream for the above-mentioned reasons. Then, especially if you have *oily* skin, try using a mild soap and water wash. The slight drying effect of most soaps could, and I think *would* be advantageous for this skin type. If you have *normal* or *dry* skin, and wish to use a soap and water wash, be sure to select only mild, pure products (preferable super-fatted with some moisturizing ingredient) and do not let the soap remain on your skin for a long period of time.

Rinse well. Unless your water is very soft, it is sometimes difficult to get all of the soap off the skin. A soap residue can lead to itching, chapping, and even infection if it's able to snag bacteria and dirt particles, which will then stay in your pores to cause trouble. So rinse well, then rinse again.

No matter how meticulous you may be, I would shy away from most soaps entirely if you have extremely dry or aging skin.   The great majority of soaps do seem to further dry the skin and that *you* do not need.

In any event, soap or no soap, you should begin with a cleansing cream.

The method of application and removal varies slightly for each skin type, so consult Chapter Five to learn your own individual routine.

Recipes for Cleansing Creams for Normal and Dry Skins

Crisco Cleansing Cream

1 can crisco

That's all.   People in the theater have been using it for years to remove their stage makeup.   It's natural hydro-genated cottonseed oil (hydrogenated oils are those which through a special treatment have been hardened).   It works beautifully and is inexpensive.   And it won't take you long to make, either.

Your Favorite Perfume Cleansing Cream

3   tbsp safflower oil
4   tsp beeswax
1   tbsp witch hazel
1   tbsp your favorite perfume or cologne
1   tbsp almond oil
1/8   tsp borax
1/2   tsp zinc oxide ointment

Melt beeswax over *low* heat.   Beat in warmed almond and safflower oil. Dissolve borax in slightly warmed witch hazel and perfume. Pour slowly, beating constantly, into oil and wax mixture. Beat until cool and then beat in zinc oxide. Makes about 3 oz. Refrigerate.

Glycerin and Rose Water Cleansing Cream

4	tbsp anhydrous lanolin
2	oz soy oil
3	tbsp rose water
1	tbsp glycerin
1	tsp zinc oxide ointment
1/8	tsp borax
1/4	tsp oil of roses (if not available use the essential oil of any flower)

Melt lanolin. Heat soy oil and glycerin and dribble into lanolin, beating constantly. Dissolve borax in rose water and beat into mixture. When cool and creamy, add zinc oxide and scented oil. Makes 4 oz. Refrigerate.

Cocoa Butter Cleansing Cream

1	oz cocoa butter
1	oz safflower oil
1	oz almond oil
1	oz rose water
1	tbsp beeswax
1/8	tsp borax

Melt beeswax over low heat. Melt cocoa butter separately and add to other warmed oils. Dribble oils into beeswax, beating constantly. Warm rose water and borax and beat into first mixture. Beat until creamy and cool. Makes 3 oz. Refrigerate.

Herbal Cleansing Cream with Almonds

1	tbsp sage
1	tbsp thyme
1	tbsp oregano
1	cup water
2	tbsp anhydrous lanolin
2	tsps spermaceti
2	tsps beeswax

2   oz sesame oil
2   oz olive oil
1/2   tsp almond extract
1/8   tsp borax
2   tbsp pulverized almonds

Boil water. Steep herbs for an hour or so. Strain and set aside. (You will be using 3 tbsp of the herb water. Try using the left-over water as a steam soup, see Chapter Four). Pulverize almonds in blender or crush with a mortar and pestle and set aside. Melt lanolin, spermaceti and beeswax over low heat. Warm oils and beat into wax mixture for 3 to 5 minutes. Dissolve borax in hot herb water and, pouring slowly, beat into mixture until creamy and cool (5 to 10 minutes). Beat in extract and almonds. When using this cream, use a washing motion to benefit from the abrasive action which will help to remove dead skin cells. Makes about 5 oz. Refrigerate.

Jiffy Fresh Fruit Cleansing Cream

6   tbsp Crisco
2   tbsp any fresh, strained fruit juice (lemon, orange, grapefruit, strawberry, etc).
1/8   tsp borax

Melt Crisco over low heat. Dissolve borax in hot fruit juice and beat into Crisco until cool and creamy. Makes 3 oz. (Don't worry if the consistency gets a little grainy; it foams up beautifully when massaged onto the face.) Refrigerate.

Avocado Cleansing Cream

3   oz avocado oil
2   tbsp fresh avocado
1   tbsp beeswax
1   tbsp anhydrous lanolin
1 1/2 tsp coconut oil
1   tsp alcohol
2   tbsp witch hazel
1/8   tsp borax

Melt beeswax and lanolin over low heat. Warm oils and beat into wax mixture. Dissolve borax in warm witch hazel and alcohol and, pouring slowly, beat into mixture until cool and creamy. Mash avocado in a small, flat dish with a fork. Push through a strainer with a fork or your fingers until you have nothing but fibers left in the strainer. Beat avocado into cream with 2 drops of green food coloring. Definitely refrigerate. Makes 4 oz.

Strawberry Liquid Cleanser

2	tbsp anhydrous lanolin
2	oz soy oil
1	tbsp plus 1 tsp strawberry extract
1/4	tsp borax
1	tbsp fresh strawberry juice

Melt lanolin over low heat. Heat soy oil and beat into lanolin. Dissolve borax in extract and, pouring very slowly, beat into mixture for at least 5 minutes. Beat in strawberry juice (if it's foamy, don't worry) and put in bottle. (This is light enough to go in a dispenser bottle). Makes 5 oz.

Simple Liquid Cleanser

Vegetable oil of your choice

That's all. If you want a scent, shake it up with 1 oz. of any scented oil and shake before each use. Refrigerate.

Recipes for Cleansing Creams for Oily Skin

Petro-Gel Cleansing Cream

1 jar petroleum jelly

That's all. Just use as you would any fancy cleansing cream.

Your Favorite Perfume Cleansing Cream

2	tbsp beeswax
3	tbsp petroleum jelly
3	oz mineral oil
2	tbsp witch hazel
2	tbsp your favorite perfume or cologne
1/8	tsp borax

Melt beeswax and petroleum jelly over low heat. Warm mineral oil and beat into wax mixture for 3 to 5 minutes. Dissolve borax in warmed witch hazel and perfume. Pour slowly into mixture, beating constantly until cool and creamy. Makes about 4 oz.

Oatmeal Cleansing Cream

2	tbsp oatmeal (not instant or 1-minute)
1	tbsp petroleum jelly
1	tbsp anhydrous lanolin
2	tsp spermaceti
2	tsp beeswax
2	oz mineral oil
1	oz castor oil
1	tbsp rose water
1/8	tsp borax

Melt petroleum jelly, spermaceti, lanolin and beeswax over low heat. Warm mineral and castor oils and beat into mixture for 3 to 5 minutes. Dissolve borax in warm rose water and beat into mixture. Continue beating for 5 to 10 minutes until soft cream is formed. (I recommend an electric beater for this one, as it takes more than usual beating.) Beat in oatmeal.

Scrub face lightly with this cream before removing it. The abrasive action helps to loosen blackheads and rids the face of dead skin cells. Makes 4 oz.

Creme de Menthe Liquid Cleanser

2   tbsp anhydrous lanolin
3   oz glycerin
1   oz mineral oil
1   oz creme de menthe extract
1/4   tsp borax

Melt lanolin over low heat. Warm glycerin and mineral oil and beat into lanolin. Dissolve borax in warmed extract and pouring slowly, beat into mixture until cool and creamy. Pour into bottle. (This is light enough to go in a dispenser bottle.) Makes 4 oz.

Jiffy Fresh Fruit Cleansing Cream

6   tbsp petroleum jelly
1   tbsp fresh, strained fruit juice (lemon, orange, grapefruit, strawberry, etc.)
1/4   tsp borax

Melt petroleum jelly over *low* heat. Dissolve borax in hot fruit juice and beat into petroleum jelly until cool and creamy. Refrigerate. Makes 3 oz.

Castile Cleansing Cream

3   tsp beeswax
1   tsp spermaceti
2   tbsp petroleum jelly
1 1/2 oz mineral oil
2   tsp coconut oil
2   tbsp rose water
1/8   tsp borax
1   tbsp shaved castile soap

Melt beeswax, spermaceti, petroleum jelly and castile soap over *very low* heat. (Don't be concerned if the soap doesn't melt completely. It will blend in when you start mixing.) Warm mineral and coconut oils together and beat into first mixture. Dissolve borax in warmed rose water and, pouring slowly, beat into mixture until cool and creamy. To use, wash face as if using soap and water; remove with wet washcloth. Makes about 4 oz.

Spiced Cleansing Gel

2   oz spiced glycerin
2   oz light mineral oil
1   tsp plain gelatin

To make spiced glycerin, place 4 or 5 coarsely crushed cinnamon sticks (or 1 to 2 tbsp crushed whole cloves, or both) in the 2 oz of glycerin. Let stand in a small glass container for a week or so until heavily scented. Strain the spiced glycerin and discard the spices. Heat glycerin with the mineral oil and dissolve the gelatin in mixture. Beat until cool and creamy. When using, remove gel with a washing motion to benefit from the slight abrasive action. Makes 4 oz.

Strawberry Cleansing Cream

1   tsp spermaceti
2   tbsp petroleum jelly
1   oz castor oil
1   oz mineral oil
1   tsp coconut oil
1   tbsp plus 1 tsp strawberry extract
1/4 tsp borax
1   tbsp fresh strawberry juice

Melt spermaceti and petroleum jelly over *low* heat. Warm oils together and beat into mixture. Dissolve borax in warm extract and beat into mixture until cool and creamy (3 to 5 minutes). Beat fresh strawberry juice (don't worry if it's foamy) into cream. Makes 4 oz. Refrigerate.

Simple Liquid Cleanser

1 bottle light mineral oil

That's all. If you want a scent, shake it up with 1 oz any scented oil and shake before each use.

Skin Fresheners

These lotions have many different names: skin toners or tonics, conditioners, astringents, cleansing lotions, fresheners, and texture lotions are a few of them. They are used after a cleansing cream for specific purposes, and the *least* important is that they make your skin feel fresh and alive. For oily skins, they're essential because they effectively remove any oils which may remain on the skin from the cleansing cream. And they are enthusiastically recommended for all skin types because they tone and freshen the skin as well as stimulate circulation to promote that all-important internal cleansing. In addition, fresheners restore the skin's pH to normal (should it be necessary) and tighten and close pores for a refined texture.

You'll hear those terms repeated time and again: "tighten pores," "close enlarged pores." Actually, none of that really happens. True "pores," which are the minute openings of sweat glands, are hidden from the naked eye. They usually reach only the border between the dermis and the epidermis.

What is commonly thought of as a "pore" on the surface of the skin is actually an opening of the follicle of a baby hair which you may or may not be able to see. Sometimes the openings grow large (naturally) in order to prepare not for a baby hair but for a large one. Then if the large hair doesn't appear for some reason, you have an enlarged "pore."

Since the misnomer is solidly ingrained in beauty vocabulary, I shall also refer to follicle openings as "pores." I just thought it would be informative to stop and point out these interesting facts.

To return to fresheners. Not only are the openings not "pores" that the lotions close and tighten, but the lotions don't "close" and "tighten" either. What actually happens is this: the slightly astringent qualities of the lotion cause the surrounding tissue to swell so that the tiny opening *seems* to be smaller or "closed" and "tightened." This gives the skin that smooth, fine-grained texture so sought after by women of all skin types.

Now that you are aware of what fresheners do and don't do, let me tell you how to apply these amazing lotions. This is best done with cottonballs.   Shake the bottle of lotion, hold the cotton over the opening until it is wet (not dripping), then, with firm movements to stimulate

APPLYING SKIN FRESHENER

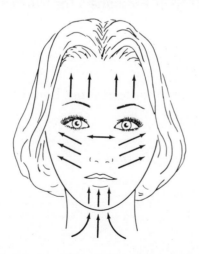

circulation, wipe the areas to be cleaned in an upward and outward motion. Use fresh cotton as needed. It's well to remember that you're not wiping the lotion *on*, you're wiping any leftover dirt *off*.

These fresheners are effective any time of the day for a quick cleanup or pick-me-up for the face. There are recipes for oily skins and dry and normal skins. If you have a combination skin, you get to use one of each.

For those of you who may be new to this type of lotion, I think you'll enjoy the spanking clean feeling it imparts to your face. *I* believe that skin fresheners are the single most important cleaning agent you can use on your face. If *you* don't believe it, put it to the test. Clean your face the way you normally do — cleansing cream, soap and water or whatever — and then, when you're absolutely sure that your skin is clean, use a skin freshener according to the above directions. I think you'll be surprised at the amount of additional dirt you find on the cotton ball. . .dirt that would have remained on your face all day if you hadn't used the skin freshener.

Recipes for Skin Fresheners for Normal Skin

Witch Hazel Lotion

1 bottle witch hazel

That's all. Just use this refreshing liquid by itself as you would any other fancier lotion.

Glycerin and Rose Water Lotion

4   oz rose water
1/2-1 oz glycerin
1   oz witch hazel

Shake together in bottle.

Barley Water Tonic

1/4 cup barley
1   qt water
1/2 cup witch hazel

In saucepan, bring barley and water to boil. Lower heat and simmer for about an hour. Strain until clear. When cool, add witch hazel, bottle and keep in refrigerator. When using, apply as usual and follow with a cold water rinse.

Orange Water Freshener

3   oz orange extract (for different scent, select different extract)
2   oz witch hazel
1/8 tsp alum

Shake together in bottle.

Gin and Tonic Freshener

1   oz good quality gin
3   oz rose water
3   oz witch hazel

Don't drink. Shake together in bottle instead.
Normal skins may also use fresheners for dry skin. See additional recipes under Dry Skin Fresheners.

Milk Cleansers for Any Type of Skin

Milk has been used as a cleanser for thousands of years. It not only cleans, but it has a slight bleaching power to keep your skin dewy *and* white. Once made, keep these cleansers in the refrigerator or you'll soon have a *sour* milk lotion which may do wonders for pancakes but not much for your face.

Apply with cotton pads and rinse face with cool water.

Cucumber Cleansing Milk

3   oz cucumber juice
3   oz milk

Shake together in bottle.

Orange or Strawberry Cleansing Milk

3   oz fresh orange or strawberry juice
3   oz milk

Shake together strained juice and milk in a bottle.

Cleansing Lotions for Dry Skin

The following recipes are beneficial to dry skin but they can all be used equally well for normal skin, too.

Lemon or Orange Freshener

1   oz fresh lemon or orange juice
1   oz lemon or orange extract
1/2-1 oz glycerin
3   oz witch hazel

Strain lemon or orange juice and shake together with remaining ingredients in bottle. Refrigerate.

Rose Water and Glycerin Freshener

4   oz rose water
1   oz glycerin

Shake together in bottle.

Witch Hazel Freshener

3   oz witch hazel
1/2-1 oz glycerin

Shake together in bottle.

Strawberry or Cucumber Freshener

3   oz fresh strawberry or cucumber juice
2   oz witch hazel
2   oz rose water
1/2-1 oz glycerin

Strain strawberry or cucumber juice and shake together with remaining ingredients in bottle. Keep in refrigerator.

Chamomile Freshener

2   oz chamomile tea
4   oz witch hazel

Shake together in bottle.

Rose 'n' Mineral Water Freshener

2   oz mineral water
3   oz rose water
1/2   oz alcohol

Shake together in bottle. (This can also be used as a face spray after applying moisturizing creams.)

Lavender Freshener

3   oz lavender water
2   oz witch hazel
1/2-1 oz glycerin

Shake together in bottle.

Skin Fresheners for Oily Skin

Gin and Tonic Freshener

3   oz good quality gin
3   oz witch hazel

Shake together in bottle. Don't drink.

Screwdriver Freshener

3   oz vodka
2   oz witch hazel
1   oz fresh orange juice
1   tbsp orange extract

Strain orange juice and shake together with other ingredients in bottle. Don't drink. Refrigerate.

Brandy Freshener

2   oz good brandy
1   oz alcohol
3   oz witch hazel

Shake together in bottle. Don't drink.

Witch Hazel Fizzy Freshener

4   oz witch hazel
1   oz rose water
1   oz alcohol
1   tbsp camphor water
1/4 tsp boric acid
1   tsp tincture of benzoin

Shake together in bottle.

Rose Water Freshener #1

3   oz rose water
1   oz witch hazel

2   oz alcohol
1/2 tsp alum

Shake together in bottle.

Rose Water Freshener #2

3   oz rose water
2   oz alcohol
3   tsp camphor water

Shake together in bottle.

Strawberry Freshener

2   oz strawberry juice
2   oz witch hazel
2   oz alcohol
1/2 tsp boric acid

Shake together in bottle. Refrigerate.

Cucumber Freshener

3   oz cucumber juice
2   oz witch hazel
2   oz rose water
1   oz alcohol

Strain cucumber juice (skin and all) and shake together with other ingredients in bottle. Refrigerate. (If you want this less perishable, peel the cucumber.)

Lemon or Grapefruit Freshener

2   oz fresh lemon or grapefruit juice
3   oz witch hazel

1   oz alcohol

1   tbsp lemon extract

Strain lemon juice and shake together with other ingredients in bottle. Refrigerate.

Moisturizing and Protection Creams

There are many names for these creams. "Moisturizing" cream is one of them, "penetrating" cream is another. The old-fashioned term is "vanishing" cream. You may have also heard "protection" cream or "replenishing" cream.

Whatever the name, the basic function is the same. To lubricate, soften, and moisturize the skin and protect it from the elements.

The moisture *every* type of skin requires is water. Experiments have shown that when chapped, dry skins were treated with oils alone the condition was not improved. However, when *water* was added or conserved in the skin, the problem was alleviated at once.

"Moisturize" in this case doesn't mean to *add* moisture. It may do that slightly by holding the water in the cream in close contact with the skin for a brief moment. But since the water evaporates immediately (that's the cool feeling you get when applying a cream of this type), the value is minimal. The greatest importance of a moisturizing or protection cream seems to be in its ability to form a light, transparent film over the skin's surface which acts as a barrier so that water being sent to the skin from the *inside* by way of the underlying tissues *doesn't* evaporate. So it's really a moisture-*retaining* cream.

Because of the previous reasons, the regular use of a moisturizing or protection cream is desirable for *all* types of skin. The unique requirements of the *individual* skin types are just that: unique and individual. And these requirements, you now know, are fulfilled by the choice of *oils* used in the making of the creams — penetrating vegetable oils to moisturize by stimulating and replenishing the natural oils of normal and dry skin and *non*penetrating mineral oils to protect the surface *without* stimulating the natural oils of oily skins. Ergo: "moisturing" creams for normal and dry skins and "protection" creams for oily skins.

Moisturizing Creams for Normal and Dry Skin

With moisturizing creams, a deep, upward and outward massage should be used. This stimulates the circulation of the blood which nourishes the skin and all its structures. In addition to that, with a deep massage the muscle fiber is stimulated and strengthened. This is important for all skins as it helps to maintain elasticity, but for aging skins it is crucial. Deep massage promotes glandular activity, specifically the sebaceous glands, and tends to reduce fat cells. Needless to say, the nerves are soothed and your skin becomes soft, fresh, and alive.

After using massaging creams (use small amounts; remember these creams are *rich*) in the suggested manner, there probably won't be a trace left to be seen on your face. If there is, simply blot it off with a clean tissue.

If you have dry skin, you may want to spray some mineral water or rose water (keep it in the refrigerator in an old, well-scrubbed Windex bottle) lightly over your face after applying the cream. It will help the cream penetrate while hydrating your skin.

For the following massage methods, use the middle and ring finger of both hands.

MASSAGE TECHNIQUES
FOR MOISTURIZING CREAMS

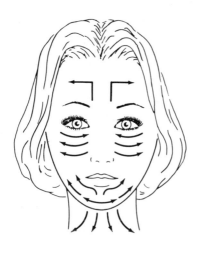
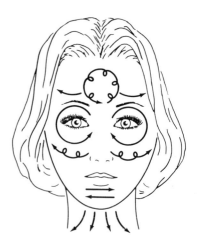

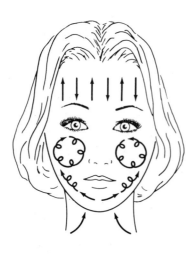
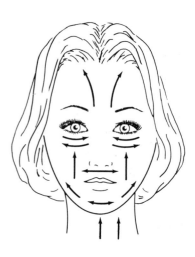

Recipes for Moisturizing Creams

Coconut-Vitamin Liquid Moisturizer

1	oz coconut extract
4	tbsp coconut oil
1/2	tsp vitamin A & D oil
2	tsp cocoa butter
2	tsp soy oil
2 1/2	tsp anhydrous lanolin
1/4	tsp borax
1/2	tsp liquid lecithin

Melt lanolin over low heat. Warm coconut oil, cocoa butter, lecithin, soy oil, and vitamin A & D oil (use in liquid form or pierce vitamin capsules and empty contents into measuring spoon) together, and beat into lanolin. Dissolve borax in warm extract and, pouring slowly, beat into mixture until cool and creamy (3 to 5 minutes). Put in bottle; this cream is light enough to go in a dispenser bottle. Makes over 4 oz.

Protein Moisturizing Cream

1	oz olive oil
2	tbsp anyhdrous lanolin
1	egg yolk
1/4	tsp orange extract
1/2	tsp liquid lecithin

Melt lanolin over low heat. Warm oil and lecithin and beat into lanolin until cool and creamy. Beat egg yolk and extract into cream until fluffy and put in jar. Definitely refrigerate. Makes 4 oz.

Cucumber Moisturizing Cream

1	tbsp beeswax
2	oz soy oil

1/2   tsp liquid lecithin
1   tbsp cucumber juice
1   tbsp witch hazel
1/8   tsp borax
3   drops green food coloring
1/2   tsp liquid lecithin

Wash cucumber thoroughly and wipe dry. Squeeze or blend (with skin on) and strain about 1 oz juice. Heat briefly, do not boil, and set aside. Melt beeswax over low heat. Warm soy oil and lecithin and, pouring slowly, beat into wax. Heat 1 tbsp of the cucumber juice with the witch hazel and borax and, pouring slowly, beat into mixture until cool and creamy. Beat in food coloring. Makes 4 oz. Refrigerate.

Tinted Moisturizing Cream

Get 1 to 2 oz of a powder called *Neutracolor* from your druggist and stir it (a little at a time) into the moisturizing cream of your choice. If the original recipe calls for food coloring, omit it. When you have achieved the desired shade, you can use the cream in place of foundation; it's a great way to go bare-faced and yet have a glow of color. You'll have to make the cream quite dark (keep testing the color on your face) as it appears much lighter when you apply it.

Blended Oils Liquid Moisturizer

1   oz almond oil
1   oz avocado oil
1   oz sesame oil
1   oz wheat germ oil
1   tsp liquid lecithin

Heat all together gently and pour into bottle. You can substitute any oils you wish, of course, I have chosen these because they are ultrarich. If you would like to have a lovely fragrance, simply substitute a scented oil in place of one of the oils. The moisturizer is especially wonderful for very dry or aging skin. (Also makes a great body lotion.) Makes 4 oz. Definitely refrigerate and shake before each use.

Vitamin A, D & E Cream with Lecithin

1	tbsp almond oil
1	tbsp avocado oil
1	tbsp wheat germ oil
1	tbsp beeswax
1/2	tsp spermaceti
1	tsp anhydrous lanolin
1	tsp cocoa butter
1 1/2	tsp liquid lecithin
1	tsp vitamin A
1/2	tsp vitamin D
1/8	tsp borax
3	oz rose water

Melt beeswax, spermaceti and lanolin over low heat. Melt cocoa butter and add to heated oils. Add lecithin to oils. Beat oil mixture into wax mixture until creamy. Heat rose water and borax and, pouring very slowly, beat into cream. Vitamin A and D capsules come in oil form. Pierce them with a pin, squeeze out the proper amount and stir into cream. Refrigerate. Makes 3 oz.

Cocoa Butter Moisturizing Cream

2	oz cocoa butter
1 1/2	oz peanut oil
1	tbsp beeswax
2	tbsp witch hazel
1	tsp liquid lecithin
1/2	tsp zinc oxide ointment
1/8	tsp borax

Melt beeswax over low heat. Melt cocoa butter and warm together with peanut oil and lecithin. Beat oil mixture into wax. Dissolve borax in warm witch hazel and, pouring slowly, beat into mixture until creamy and cool. Beat in zinc oxide and put in jar. Makes 3 oz. Refrigerate.

Honey-Lemon Liquid Moisturizer

3   tbsp anhydrous lanolin
2   tsp cocoa butter
1   tsp coconut oil
1   tbsp safflower oil
1   tsp honey
1   oz lemon oil
1/2   tsp liquid lecithin

Melt lanolin and cocoa butter over low heat. Add honey. Warm coconut oil, lecithin, and safflower oil and, pouring slowly, beat into first mixture. Beat in lemon oil until creamy and cool and put in jar or bottle. Makes 4 oz. Refrigerate.

APPLYING PROTECTION CREAM

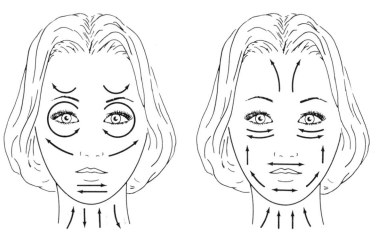

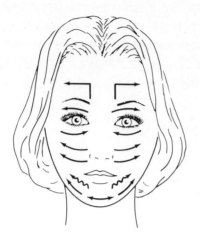

Protection Creams for Oily Skin

A deep massage is not for oily skins. Stimulation of overzealous oil glands would only add to your troubles.

Smooth a dab of protection cream over the face with upward and outward movements until you are assured of light coverage, not "smotherage"; *small amounts only* are necessary. The movements should be firm and decisive to stimulate circulation of the blood which will in turn oxygenate and feed the skin. It will also tone the underlying muscles slightly to help preserve the elasticity of the skin. Don't let it turn into a massage, however; it would surely excite your sebaceous glands and extend your already-existing problem.

Blot off any excess cream.

Recipes for Protection Creams

Scented Protection Cream

4	tsp beeswax
4	tsp spermaceti
2	oz light mineral oil
2	tbsp favorite scent (almond is lovely) extract
1/8	tsp borax

Melt beeswax and spermaceti over low heat. Warm mineral oil and beat into wax mixture. Dissolve borax in warm extract and pouring slowly beat into mixture until cool and creamy. Makes over 4 oz. (To make unscented, substitute witch hazel for extract.)

Cucumber Protection Cream

1	tbsp cucumber juice
1	tbsp witch hazel
2	oz mineral oil
1	tbsp beeswax
1/4	tsp borax
2	drops green food coloring

Wash cucumber thoroughly and wipe dry. Squeeze or blend and strain about 2 oz into a small pan and heat briefly. (Do not boil.) Set aside. Melt beeswax over low heat. Warm oil and beat into wax. Dissolve borax in 1 tbsp heated cucumber juice and the witch hazel and, pouring slowly, beat into first mixture until cool and creamy. Beat in food coloring. Makes 4 oz.

Rose 'n' Glycerin Protection Fluid

2	oz rose water
2	oz glycerin

Shake together in bottle. Shake before each use. Makes 4 oz.

Tinted Protection Cream

Get an ounce or two of a powder called *Neutracolor* from your druggist. Stir it (in small amounts) into the protection cream of your choice. If the original cream called for food coloring, omit it. When the desired shade is achieved, you can use your cream in place of a foundation on those days you wish to go barefaced but have a glow. You have to make the cream quite dark (keep checking the color by smoothing it on your face as you color along) as it lightens when applied.

Lemon Protection Cream

2	tbsp mineral oil
2	tbsp anhydrous lanolin
3	tbsp petroleum jelly
1	tbsp fresh lemon juice
1	oz lemon extract
1/4	tsp borax

4 to 6 drops yellow food coloring

Melt lanolin and petroleum jelly over *low* heat. Warm mineral oil and beat into mixture. Heat lemon juice, extract, and borax and, pouring slowly, beat into cream mixture. Beat until cool and creamy. Beat in food coloring and put in jar. Makes 3 oz. Refrigerate.

Protein Protection Cream

1	tbsp beeswax
1	tsp spermaceti
1	oz coconut oil
1	oz mineral oil
1	tsp alcohol
2	tbsp rose water (scant measure)
1/8	tsp borax
1	egg yolk

Melt beeswax and spermaceti over low heat. Heat coconut and mineral oil and beat into wax mixture. Dissolve borax in rose water and alcohol and, pouring slowly, beat into mixture until cool and creamy. Beat in egg yolk. Makes 3 oz. Definitely refrigerate.

Herbal Protection Cream

1   tbsp beeswax
1   tbsp spermaceti
2   oz mineral oil
1   oz castor oil
2   tbsp herb water (see recipe below)
1/8 tsp borax

To make herb water steep 1 1/2 tsp each dried sage and oregano leaves in 3 oz boiled water. Strain after 10 minutes and set aside. Melt beeswax and spermaceti over low heat. Warm oils and beat into waxes. Heat 2 tbsp of the herb water with the borax and, pouring slowly, beat into mixture. Beat until cool and creamy. Makes just under 5 oz.

Scented Protection Fluid

1   tbsp petroleum jelly
1   oz light mineral oil
2   oz scented oil of your choice
1/4 tsp boric acid
1   oz witch hazel

Melt petroleum jelly over *very low* heat. Warm mineral oil, turn off heat and add scented oil. Beat oils into petroleum jelly. Dissolve boric acid in witch hazel and, pouring slowly, beat into mixture. Beat for 4 to 5 minutes until cool and creamy. Pour into a bottle and shake before each use. Makes over 3 oz.

3

Cream Pies for the Eyes

The face is the mirror of the mind, and eyes without speaking confess the secrets of the heart.

—St. Jerome

Your eyes. As delicate and precious as the soul they express. Not only do they see, but they allow your Self to be seen. Is it any wonder we pamper and pat them, cool and refresh them, and take it to heart each time a new wrinkle surrounds them?

The hard facts are these: there are no oil glands around the eye area. The skin is very thin and gets little, if any, circulation. Which all adds up to wrinkles and premature aging.

An eye cream, consequently, serves an entirely different function from any other type of moisturizing cream. Since there are no sebaceous glands to stimulate, we have no need for the penetrating powers of natural vegetable oils. As a matter of fact, each eye moisturizer in this chapter is specifically designed *not* to penetrate. There are several reasons for this.

One of the purposes in applying a moisturizer to the eye area is to lubricate. If those little crinkles and lines surrounding the eyes are kept moist, they won't deepen as quickly. Lines cannot be stopped, but they can be retarded to an amazing degree. If you were to stop smiling, that would also help, but then you

TO APPLY EYE CREAM

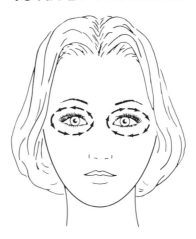

USE YOUR MIDDLE FINGER AND MAKE TWO OR THREE LITTLE CIRCLES AT THE OUTER CORNER (WHERE WRINKLES ARE USUALLY MORE PREVALENT) AND THEN CONTINUE TOWARD THE INNER CORNER OF THE EYE AND ON AROUND.

couldn't call them "laugh lines" and who would recommend that anyway? Not I.

Because it's helpful to keep the skin around the eyes lubricated at all times, each recipe includes oils that will not penetrate.

Another purpose of an eye cream or gel is to attempt to soften the skin and actually diminish the appearance of lines. There are certain oils — such as castor oil, cocoa butter, and coconut oil — which have been shown to contain properties which accomplish this. I'm not saying that creams made with these oils will *erase* lines and wrinkles. No beauty aid discovered or created so far has that magical power and don't ever let anyone tell you it has. What eye gels do have the power to do, however, is to soften the area and therefore erase the sharp appearance of the lines.

A caution here about makeup. Many women who cleanse and moisturize their skin properly proceed unknowingly to undo all of the goodness with makeup. When you apply it, use as little as possible on any area which is lined. *Never* apply makeup *directly* to the wrinkles. Rather, using your fingertips in a patting motion, blend under-eye makeup into the rest of your foundation. Never, *ever*, apply powder or dry blushers to a wrinkled skin. It only deepens the crevices.

During the day when you freshen your makeup, tap a "crinkle stick" (recipe included) gently over the eye area to relubricate it. You'll notice a tremendous difference immediately when you keep this delicate eye area moist with softening, nonpenetrable creams and gels.

And that's all you can do. So do it. And forget it. Many people, and I'm one of them, think that "laugh lines" are lovely. . .on both men and women. But if they bother you, I think the most constructive and realistic thing to remember is that other people aren't looking at your *lines*, they're looking into your *eyes*. It's what they read there, between the lines, as it were, that makes the difference.

Recipes

The Wrinkle Arrester

3	tbsp anhydrous lanolin
5	tsp coconut oil
3	tsp olive oil
1	tbsp mineral oil
3	oz castor oil

Melt lanolin and coconut oil together. Heat olive, mineral and castor oils in separate pan. Pour oils slowly into lanolin mixture, beating constantly. Beat until cream thickens. Makes approximately 5 oz.

Coconut Butter Cream

2   oz mineral oil
2   tbsp coconut oil
2   tbsp cocoa butter

Heat together and beat until cool. Makes about 3 3/4 oz.

Almond Eye Cream

1   oz plus 1 tbsp almond oil
1   oz plus 1 tbsp castor oil
2   tsp anhydrous lanolin
2   tbsp mineral oil
2   tsp beeswax
pinch sodium benzoate

Over low heat, melt beeswax and lanolin. Warm the oils in separate pan. Add sodium benzoate to oils and pour mixture into wax mixture. Beat until cool. Makes a little under 4 oz.

Avocado Cream

2   tbsp avocado oil
2   oz castor oil
2   tbsp petroleum jelly
2   tbsp anhydrous lanolin

Heat lanolin and petroleum jelly together over low heat. Warm oils and add slowly, beating all the while, to the lanolin mixture. Beat until cool. Makes a little over 4 oz.

Baby Balm

1 1/2 oz mineral oil
1 1/2 oz castor oil
3   tbsp anhydrous lanolin

3   tsp cocoa butter
3   tsp coconut oil
2   tbsp petroleum jelly

Heat lanolin and petroleum jelly over low heat. Heat liquid oils, cocoa butter, and coconut oil and beat into lanolin mixture. Beat until cool. Makes 5 oz.

Ultrarich Eye Gel

2   tbsp petroleum jelly
2   tbsp cocoa butter
2   tbsp coconut oil
2   tbsp anhydrous lanolin

Heat lanolin and petroleum jelly over low heat. Heat cocoa butter and coconut oil together and beat into lanolin mixture. Beat until cool. Makes approximately 3 oz.

Vitamin E Cream for the Eyes

1   oz mineral oil
1   oz wheat germ oil
1   tbsp coconut oil
1   tbsp anhydrous lanolin
2   tsp beeswax

Melt beeswax and lanolin over low heat. Warm oils and beat into wax mixture until cool. Makes about 3 oz.

Crinkle Sticks

When you have finished preparing one of these crinkle stick creams, rotate the bottom of a well-scrubbed, dry lipstick case until the inside portion reaches the top. Use fingers to pack the cream into the case, pressing down firmly. When the cream is filled to the top, rotate the

the bottom of the tube downward to allow more room for
further packing. Continue this process until the tube is
filled. To apply, simply tap lightly onto wrinkled area.

Cocoa Butter Crinkle Stick

1   oz cocoa butter
1   tsp spermaceti
1   tsp heavy mineral oil

Melt cocoa butter and spermaceti over low heat. Beat in
warmed mineral oil and continue beating until cool.
Scoop into two lipstick cases.

Slick Crinkle Stick

1   tbsp petroleum jelly
1/2   tsp anhydrous lanolin
1   tsp beeswax
1/2   tsp spermaceti
1   tbsp cocoa butter

Melt first four ingredients over low heat. Melt cocoa
butter and beat into first mixture. Beat until cool and
scoop into two lipstick cases.

Beeswax Crinkle Stick

1   tsp beeswax
1   tsp petroleum jelly
1/2   tsp anhydrous lanolin

Melt all together over low heat and beat until cool.
Scoop into two lipstick cases.

Waxy Beeswax Crinkle Stick

2   tsp beeswax
1/2   tsp spermaceti
2   tsp petroleum jelly
1   tsp anhydrous lanolin

Melt all four ingredients over low heat and beat until cool. Scoop into two lipstick cases.

4

Menus for a Masked Ball

*Creating from themselves, all beauties
are Creators of the beautiful.*
—E.H. Burrington

There are many valid reasons for applying a weekly beauty mask. The mask can tighten your skin and minimize pore size; it can bleach; it can penetrate and moisturize; it can act as a superficial peeler to rid the face of accumulated dead skin cells. If the ingredients used in the mask contain protein, it can even possibly repair superficially damaged skin. Whichever mask you choose, for whatever purpose, there's one thing they all do, and that is to *deeply cleanse*, soften, and bring to life a rosy, silky skin that has nothing to hide.

Deep cleansing stimulates circulation and draws the blood to the surface, which oxygenates or feeds the skin and also causes the internal cleansing that I discussed in Chapter One. It is the elimination of impurities *beneath* the surface of the skin that causes the surface to glow.

If you are faithful to a weekly or biweekly beauty mask, your cleansing creams and skin fresheners and your moisturizers will be able to effectively maintain a dewy complexion on all of your unmasked days.

You can, of course, purchase packaged beauty masks at the store, and they are certainly adequate. But nothing can duplicate the fresh, natural benefits, and the inexpensiveness of a mask *custom-made* for your own individual skin. . .right out of your refrigerator.

62

Making your own masks, as with all homemade cosmetics, also gives you allergy control. It's possible – not probable – to have an allergic reaction to even natural ingredients, but since you know what those ingredients *are* you can eliminate them one by one until you discover the one that doesn't like you. If you are susceptible to this annoyance, it surely is easier (and *cheaper*) to hop from one ingredient to another in your supermarket than to hop from one brand to another in your department store.

Tips for Applying Beauty Masks

Always apply a beauty mask to a clean face. That means removing all makeup with a cleansing cream first, then swiping away every last trace of dirt and grime with the skin freshener of your choice.

After cleansing, you may want to start your minifacial with a relaxing and beneficial steam bath for your face. The warmth of the steam opens the pores, unclogs them, and encourages toxins to be eliminated externally. . .all of which is necessary for the hygiene of your skin.

I do not recommend *dry* heat, however. It does cause the skin to perspire and eliminate impurities. That's good. It can also cause the skin to become dehydrated. That's bad. Water is one of the most precious commodities the skin requires, and it's not a wise idea to get rid of too much of it on purpose. Steam heat offers the gentle calor necessary to purge the system of poisons and at the same time surrounds the skin with hydrating water particles.

That's *gentle* heat. Never subject your skin to HOT *anything* unless you wish to relax the elasticity of your skin right along with your spirit.

A ten-minute steam with one of the steam soups from the recipe section should serve you beautifully. There are a couple of ways to go about it.

If you have a vaporizer (there are some manufactured especially for this purpose), simply add your homemade soup in the prescribed amount and steam away (unless your vaporizer specifically recommends only the use of plain water). If you're sans modern contraption, do it the way Grandma did. Heat the soup in a pot, remove from heat, and cover your head (and entire opening of the vessel) with a towel to keep the steam in. It's easy either way.

Next, pat your glowing visage dry with a soft towel and cover it all up with the mask which you have prepared in advance. And now, let me prepare *you* in advance. Beauty masks are beautifying things, *but* they are also "messifying" things. I suggest you wear nothing at all from the waist up; then, if a strawberry slips from your nose to your shoulder, you can just pop it in your mouth. However, if you must wear something, make it a plastic cape or an old towel pinned around your shoulder. . .and nothing that can't be thrown in the wash under that. Like your body.

Pin your hair up and keep the little wisps away from your face with a turban or a headband.

A man's shaving brush is a nice, professional method of applying the soupier masks, but your fingers are harder to misplace and they work just as well.

If your skin is extremely thin or sensitive, stay away from the abrasive masks — like the ones containing oatmeal or almonds — and the strong pulling masks — such as egg white, or mint. Do not apply masks over an open wound and, in all cases, do not cover the eye area with the mask. Dab some honey (a good natural moisturizer) under your eyes while the mask is on your face.

Once you have your mask on, you are free to do anything you can dream up for the ten to twenty minutes it should remain on your face. You can lie down and rest; put your head on a towel, place cotton pads soaked in witch hazel or rose water over your eyes, and relax. You can do your nails, read a book, balance your checking account, or watch your favorite TV program. You can enjoy a snack at the same time by just taking a lick at your mask every so often.

If beauty masks are a new phenomenon to you, treat yourself to two a week for a couple of months. After that, one a week may suffice, but in the beginning the extra activity will wake up your face and let it know you mean to keep it awake. You'll see smooth "glowy" results sooner if you start off strong.

After removing the mask, check your face carefully for any black- or whiteheads lurking near the surface. *Caution must be taken when emptying clogged pores.* Take a tissue and tear it in half. Cover both index fingers and press gently but firmly on either side of the blemish. Only remove that infection which dislodges without effort. *Do not apply great pressure.* Re-cover the fingers with a clean section of the tissue for each separate re-moval. (Do not squeeze any sort of blemish on the nose. If done improperly and infection ensues, it can drain directly to the brain and prove fatal. If you have persis-tent bumps on the nose, see a dermatologist.)

When the face is clean, wipe it gently with a cotton pad moistened with witch hazel or your regular skin freshener to disinfect the area. If you have an actual eruption (as opposed to tiny imperfections hiding just under the skin which are easily removed) do not apply cream or makeup of any sort to it. If you wish to cover it with a drying agent to aid the healing process, check Chapter Six for suggestions.

Any minor impurities will be coaxed to the surface by the drawing power of the mask. If you're persistent in the regular application of a mask, I think you'll find that even these will eventually diminish if not disappear altogether.

Beauty masks are important. It's the deep cleansing they can afford your skin that assures its health. . .and resulting beauty.

Your face is subjected to more smog, dirt, fumes, and direct heat and cold than any other part of your body. Not to mention the chemicals and impure substances applied, *on purpose*, in the form of makeup.

None of this is formidable or impossible to deal with. These conditions make it difficult perhaps, but a clean, silky, beautiful skin can still be yours. It just takes a little extra effort.

And beauty masks help. They may be a mess, but they're a must, so have some fun with them.

Steam Soups and Beauty Masks for Oily Skin

You will find the effective properties in each ingredient enumerated so you can mix and match recipes or substitute whatever similar food you happen to have in the house. You'll notice that most masks for oily skin emphasize 1) pulling power, which brings clogged oils to the surface as well as stimulating circulation, and 2) astringent qualities, which "tighten and close" the enlarged pores that usually accompany oily skin. The steam soups, of course, are used mostly to open the pores so the following mask can clean deeply.

Recipes for Steam Soups

Sage Soup (astringent, pore opener)

Place a handful of dried sage leaves in 1 quart of boiling water. Let steep for a couple of hours. Bring to boil again, remove from heat, and steam face for ten minutes. Leftover soup can be stored in the refrigerator and reused.

Thyme Soup (astringent, pore opener)

Use either fresh or dried thyme and follow Sage Soup recipe.

Mint Soup (pulling power, astringent, pore opener)

Use either fresh or dried mint leaves and follow Sage Soup recipe.

Recipes for Beauty Masks for Oily Skin

Almond-Cucumber Scrub

3-4   tbsp pulverized almonds (skin softener, protein, abrasive action)
1/2   freshly squeezed cucumber (astringent)

Pulverize almonds in blender or mash fine and remove oil with a paper towel. Wash cucumber well and wipe dry. Squeeze or blend cucumber (skin and all), strain it, and add in small amounts at a time to almond meal until a spreadable paste is formed. Apply to face. Leave for twenty minutes and remove with warm water followed with a splash of cold. As you remove mask, use a "washing" motion to benefit from the abrasiveness of the almonds.

Lemon-Oat Scrub

3-4 tbsp oatmeal (protein, abrasive action, vehicle for juice)
juice of one or two lemons (astringent)

Pulverize oatmeal (not instant) in blender or mash fine.   Strain lemon juice and add to oatmeal in small amounts until a spreadable paste is formed.   Apply to face. Leave for twenty minutes and remove with warm water followed with a splash of cold.   As you remove the mask, use a "washing" motion to benefit from the abrasiveness of the oatmeal.

Clay Pack

2   oz fuller's earth (pulling power, drying qualities)
2   tbsp tincture of benzoin (antiseptic)
mineral water (skin softener)

Add tincture of benzoin to fuller's earth and work in enough water to form a soft clay. Apply to face and let remain for twenty minutes. Remove with warm water followed with cold.

Strawberry Mask

3-4   tbsp bran (skin softener)
1/4   cup fresh strawberry juice (astringent)

Pulverize bran in blender or mash fine. Strain strawberry juice and blend into bran. Apply to face and let remain for twenty minutes. Rinse away with warm and then cool water.

Grapefruit Pack

2   oz fuller's earth (pulling power, drying qualities)
grapefruit juice (astringent)

Squeeze and strain fresh grapefruit. Add in small amounts to fuller's earth until a spreadable paste is formed. Apply to face and let remain for twenty minutes. Remove with warm water followed with a splash of cold.

Lemon 'n' Egg Mask

1   egg white (tightening power)
juice of 1 lemon (astringent)

Whip egg white until frothy. Beat in lemon juice. Apply to face. As first application begins to dry, add another layer. If skin is exceptionally oily, add a third layer when second is dry. Let remain on face for ten to fifteen minutes. Remove with cool water. (Leftover mask can be held in refrigerator and reused.)

Fresh Orange Mask

3-4   tbsp brewer's yeast (vitamin B, vehicle for juice, abrasive action)
juice of 1/2 orange (astringent)
1/4   tsp tincture of benzoin (antiseptic)

Mix yeast with strained orange juice to make a rather thick paste. Blend in tincture of benzoin. Apply to face and let remain for twenty minutes. Remove with warm water followed with a splash of cold. As you remove mask, use a "washing" motion to benefit from the abrasiveness of the yeast.

Tomato Mask

2   oz fresh or canned tomato juice (astringent)
2   tbsp sage leaves (astringent)
2   tbsp wheat germ (protein, vehicle for juice)

Mix ingredients together and apply to face. Let remain for twenty minutes and remove with warm and then cool water.

Rose and Almond Scrub

3-4   tbsp pulverized almonds (skin softener, protein, abrasive action)
rose water (skin softener)
1/2   tsp tincture of benzoin (antiseptic)

Blend enough rose water into the almonds to form a spreadable paste. Add tincture of benzoin. Apply to face and let remain for twenty minutes. Remove with warm water and follow with a splash of cold. When removing mask, use a "washing" motion to benefit from the abrasiveness of the almonds.

Strawberry-Mint Mask

2   oz fresh strawberry juice (astringent)
3   tbsp dried mint leaves (pulling power)
1   tbsp whole wheat flour (protein, vehicle for juice)

Blend ingredients together and apply to face. Leave on for fifteen to twenty minutes and remove with warm water followed with a splash of cold.

Steam Soups and Beauty Masks for Normal and Dry Skins

You will find the effective properties in each ingredient enumerated so you can mix and match recipes or substitute whatever similar food — including oils — you happen to have in the house. You'll notice that most masks for normal and dry skins emphasize skin softening and moisturizing, which are the specific needs of these skin types.

Recipes for Steam Soups

Chamomile Soup (skin softener, pore opener)

Use chamomile flowers or tea (or six tea bags) and add a handful to 1 quart of boiling water. Let steep a couple of hours. Bring to second boil, remove from heat, and steam face for ten minutes. Leftover soup can be stored in the refrigerator and reused.

Rose Soup (skin softener, pore opener)

Use either fresh or dried rose petals and follow Chamomile Soup recipe.

Rosemary Soup (skin softener, pore opener)

Use dried rosemary leaves and follow Chamomile Soup recipe.

Recipes for Beauty Masks

Sour Cream Mask

sour cream (skin softener, bleach)

That's all. Massage into skin and leave on for twenty minutes. Remove with warm water and follow with a splash of cold. (Plain yogurt can be substituted.)

Honey 'n' Egg Mask

1   egg (protein, pulling power)
1   tbsp honey (pulling power, moisturizer)

Whip egg until thick. Add honey and whip until blended. Apply to face and let remain for ten minutes. Remove with cool water. (Can be held in refrigerator and re-whipped at later date.)

Banana Mask

1   banana (moisturizer)
2   tbsp warm olive oil (deep penetrating moisturizer)

Mash banana and blend with oil until you have a spreadable paste. Apply to face and let remain for twenty minutes. Remove with warm water and follow with a splash of cold.

Wax Pack

2   tbsp anhydrous lanolin (moisturizer)
1   tbsp beeswax (skin softener, pulling power)
1   tbsp spermaceti (skin softener, pulling power)

Rub lanolin onto face. (Avoid eye area.) Melt waxes together, let cool slightly and apply over lanolin base. Leave on for fifteen minutes and peel off or scrape off with butter knife. Rinse face with very warm water and remove rest of mask with hot, wet washcloth.

Rose Water and Glycerin Scrub

2   tbsp rose water (skin softener)
1   tbsp glycerin (lubricator)
3-4   tbsp pulverized oatmeal (protein, abrasive action)

Pulverize oatmeal in blender or mash fine. Add rose water and glycerin small amounts at a time, until a spreadable paste is formed. Apply to face and let remain for twenty minutes. Remove with warm water and splash with cold. When removing mask, use a "washing" motion to benefit from the abrasiveness of the oatmeal.

Deep Penetrating Hot Oil Mask

Especially wonderful for very dry or aging skins.

1/2   cup virgin olive oil (moisturizer)
1   square cheesecloth

Cut out a mask from cheesecloth to fit face, leaving holes for the eyes and mouth. Warm the olive oil and soak cloth in it. Wring out lightly and fit onto face. As cloth cools, dip again into warm oil and reapply. Repeat several times. Rinse oil off face with warm water and pat dry. A nice, dewy coating will remain to protect you.

Butter-Almond Scrub

3-4 tbsp finely pulverized almonds (skin softener, protein, abrasive action)
2 tbsp margarine (moisturizer)

Pulverize almonds in blender or mash finely. Melt margarine and add in small amounts to almond meal to form a spreadable paste. Apply to face and leave on for twenty minutes. Remove with warm water followed with a splash of cold. When removing mask, use a "washing" motion to benefit from the abrasiveness of the almonds.

Avocado Mask

1/2 fresh avocado (protein, moisturizer)

Mash and heat over water until warm. Apply to face and let remain for twenty minutes. Remove with warm water and follow with a splash of cold.

Peach Mask

1 fresh, ripe peach (moisturizer)
2 tbsp peach kernel oil (moisturizer)

Peel peach and mash. Warm oil and blend into fruit until a spreadable paste is formed. Apply to face and let remain for fifteen minutes. Remove with warm and then cool water.

Mayonnaise Mask

mayonnaise (skin softener, moisturizer)

That's all. Rub it in and leave on as long as you like. Rinse with warmish water and pat dry.

Beauty Masks for any Type Skin

Protein Mask

1   egg yolk (protein, tightening power)

Whip until pale yellow and thick. Apply and leave on for ten minutes. Remove with coolish water and pat face dry.

Honey Mask

your favorite honey (pulling power, moisturizer)

That's all. Just rub into skin and let remain for twenty minutes. Remove with warm water and follow with a splash of cold.

Milk Mask

1   pack dried skim milk (skin softener, bleach)
skim milk (same properties)

Blend enough liquid skim milk with the dried milk to form a spreadable paste. Apply to face and let remain for twenty minutes. Remove with tepid water and follow with a splash of cold.

Egg White Mask

1   egg white (tightening power)

Whip until very frothy. Apply to face and let remain five to fifteen minutes. After the first layer has dried, *oily skins* can take a second and third layer. Remove with cool water. Leftover mask can be held in refrigerator, rewhipped, and reused.

Honey and Almond Scrub

3 to 4 tbsp pulverized almonds (protein, skin softener, abrasive
    action)
2   tbsp honey (pulling power, moisturizer)

Pulverize almonds in blender or mash fine. Add honey to make a thick paste. Spread on face and let remain for twenty minutes. Remove with warm water and splash with cold. When removing mask, use a "washing" motion to benefit from the abrasiveness of the almonds.

Buttermilk Pack

2   oz buttermilk (skin softener, bleach)
2   tbsp whole wheat flour or wheat germ (protein, vehicle for
    milk)

Blend milk and flour into thick paste and apply to face. Leave on for twenty minutes and remove with warm water followed with a splash of cold.

Fruit-Protein Mask

3 to 4 tbsp protein powder (protein)
your choice of fresh strawberry, grapefruit, orange, or lemon juice
    (astringents)

Add enough juice to protein powder to make spreadable paste. Apply to face. Leave on for twenty minutes and remove with warm water followed with a splash of cold.

Mint Mask

2   tbsp dried mint (astringent, pulling power)
1   cup water
1   pkg plain gelatin (protein)

Boil water and steep mint leaves for fifteen minutes. Strain liquid, reheat, and dissolve gelatin in it. While still warm, apply to face with fingers or brush. (*Oily skins* can take second or third applications.) Let remain on face for ten to fifteen minutes and remove with warm water followed with a splash of cold. Leftover mask can be jelled in refrigerator. Simply scoop out enough for one application and heat until dissolved.

Superficial Peelers for any Type Skin

This type of beauty mask can be especially beneficial if your skin is sluggish and does not regularly slough off its dead layer of skin cells. Very often that "pasty" look comes from nothing more exotic than the tenaciousness of this layer. As soon as the dead skin cells are removed, the delightful surprise of a fresh, young-looking skin is immediately discernible.

Superficial peelers can be used with great success once every couple of months (or oftener, if you like). Simply substitute one of them for a regular beauty mask during your facial.

Papaya Peeler

1/4   papaya

Mash the fresh papaya with a fork and apply to face. The enzymes in the fruit sort of "eat up" the dead layer of skin and you emerge rosy and shining.

Oatmeal Peeler

1   cup oatmeal (not instant or one-minute)

Pulverize meal in blender or mash fine and put in large bowl. Holding face over bowl, scoop oatmeal up in your hands and "dry wash" face. The abrasive action of the meal effectively removes the dead skin layer.

Salt Peeler

1/4   cup table salt

Wet washcloth with warm water. Sprinkle with salt and work slightly into cloth. Wet face with warm water. Gently scrub face with washcloth — one area at a time, avoiding eye area completely — until soft, smooth and glowing. *Do not rub hard*, this is a very effective peeler but must be used with care.

5

The Antiwrinkle Routine

*A beautiful woman is the hell of the soul,
the purgatory of the purse, and the para-
dise of the eye.*

—*Le Boyer de Fontenelle*

Now that you know how to prepare all of the separate concoctions to care for your face, it might be helpful to outline some regular beauty routines for you.

Once you get into the habit, it won't require more than ten minutes a day, and the results will be well worth it. The important thing is to establish the habit. Morning and night. *Every* morning and *every* night. More often of course if you wish, but at least make it a policy to thorougily cleanse and moisturize your face upon rising in the morning and before retiring at night.

In order to care for your skin properly, you should apply a beauty mask once a week for normal and dry skins and at least once or twice a week for oily skins.

Then add to that a monthly facial and you have the entire "antiwrinkle" routine. If you would like to apply a superfical peeler, do it in place of the beauty mask when you give yourself the complete facial.

Although the general guidelines are fundamentally the same for all skin types, there are some obvious and crucial differences. Because of that, the individual beauty routines are listed separately under skin types. Find your type and you're on your way.

Antiwrinkle Routines for Normal Skin

Morning Routine

1. Smooth cleansing cream over face. Massage well and remove with several tissues *or* rinse face with warm water and remove cream with wet, warm washcloth.
2. This step is optional, but if you want to wash with soap and water, now is the time.
3. With short, firm strokes upward and outward, cleanse entire face with cotton pads moistened with skin freshener. Use fresh cotton as needed until pad is free of dirt.
4. Apply moisturizing cream and massage deeply.
5. Apply eye cream.
6. Blot off any excess cream.
7. Apply makeup as desired.

Midday Touchup

1. Keep "crinkle stick" in your bag and when you repair your makeup pat the stick gently over any wrinkled area (right over makeup). . .around the eyes, mouth, etc.
2. Blot off any grime with a tissue lightly moistened with warm water.

Evening Routine

1. Apply cleansing cream over entire face and throat. Gently but firmly remove makeup with several clean tissues.
2. Apply cleansing cream for a second time and remove as usual.
3. Optional wash with soap and water.
4. Remove any remaining dirt or makeup with skin freshener.

5. Apply moisturizing cream and massage face thoroughly.
6. Apply eye cream.

Weekly Routine

1. Cleanse face as usual with cleansing cream.
2. Optional wash with soap and water.
3. Follow with skin freshener.
4. Steam face for ten minutes.
5. Apply beauty mask of your choice and leave on for amount of time specified in recipe.
6. Remove mask and rinse face thoroughly. Pat dry.
7. Apply moisturizing cream. Massage deeply.
8. Apply eye cream.
9. Blot off excess cream.

Monthly Facial

1. Cleanse face as usual with cleansing cream.
2. Optional wash with soap and water.
3. Follow with skin freshener.
4. Apply moisturizing cream to face. Massage thoroughly.
5. Cover face with warm, wet washcloth and lie down to rest for ten minutes.
6. Remove cream with skin freshener.
7. Steam face for ten minutes. Pat dry.
8. Apply beauty mask of your choice. Place cotton pads soaked in rose water or witch hazel over eyes.
9. Lie down and rest for specified time.
10. Remove mask and rinse face thoroughly. Pat dry.
11. Apply moisturizing cream. Massage deeply.
12. Apply eye cream.
13. Blot off excess cream.

Antiwrinkle Routines for Dry Skin

Morning Routine

1. Smooth cleansing cream over face. Massage well. Place warm, wet washcloth over face two or three times. Remove cream with washcloth.
2. This step is optional but if you want to wash with soap and water, now is the time.
3. With short, firm strokes upward and outward, cleanse entire face with cotton pads moistened in skin freshener. Use fresh cotton as needed and cleanse until pad is free of dirt.
4. Apply moisturizing cream and massage deeply.
5. Apply eye cream.
6. Blot off excess cream.
7. Spray face lightly with mineral water and let dry naturally.
8. Apply oil-based or cream makeup as desired.

Midday Touchup

1. Keep "crinkle stick" in your bag and when you repair your makeup pat the stick gently over any wrinkled area (right over makeup). . .around the eyes, mouth, etc.
2. Blot off any grime with a tissue lightly moistened with warm water.

Evening Routine

1. Apply cleansing cream over entire face. Gently but firmly remove makeup with several clean tissues.
2. Apply cleansing cream for a second time and remove as usual.
3. Optional wash with soap and water.

4. Remove any remaining dirt or makeup with skin freshener.
5. Apply moisturizing cream and massage face thoroughly.
6. Apply eye cream.
7. Blot off excess cream.
8. Spray face lightly with mineral water and let dry naturally.

Weekly Routine

1. Cleanse face as usual with cleansing cream.
2. Optional wash with soap and water.
3. Follow with skin freshener.
4. Apply moisturizing cream and eye cream.
5. Steam face for five to ten minutes.
6. Remove cream with skin freshener.
7. Apply beauty mask of your choice and leave on for amount of time specified in recipe.
8. Remove mask and rinse face thoroughly. Pat dry.
9. Apply moisturizing cream. Massage deeply.
10. Apply eye cream.
11. Blot off excess cream.
12. Spray face lightly with mineral water and let dry naturally.

Monthly Facial

1. Cleanse face as usual with cleansing cream.
2. Optional wash with soap and water.
3. Follow with skin freshener.
4. Apply eye cream.
5. Apply moisturizing cream to entire face and throat (including eye area, over eye cream).   Massage thoroughly.
6. Steam face for five to ten minutes.

7. Remove creams with skin freshener.
8. Apply warm vegetable oil of your choice to entire face and throat.
9. Cover face with warm, wet washcloth and lie down to rest for ten minutes.
10. Remove oil with skin freshener.
11. Apply beauty mask of your choice. Place cotton pads soaked in rose water or witch hazel over eyes.
12. Lie down and rest for specified time.
13. Remove mask and rinse face thoroughly. Pat dry.
14. Pat skin freshener smartly onto face with fingertips. Slap-pat repeatedly until face is dry.
15. Apply moisturizing cream. Massage deeply.
16. Apply eye cream.
17. Blot off excess cream.
18. Spray face lightly with mineral or rose water and let dry naturally.

Antiwrinkle Routines for Oily Skin

Morning Routine

1. Lay several applications of warm, wet washcloth over face to open pores.
2. Smooth cleansing cream over face. Remove with washcloth.
3. With mild soap wash face thoroughly. Rinse well and pat dry.
4. With short, firm strokes upward and outward, cleanse entire face with cotton pads moistened with skin freshener. Use fresh cotton as needed and cleanse until pad is free of dirt.
5. Apply protection cream lightly. Do not massage.
6. Apply eye cream.
7. Completely blot off excess cream.
8. Apply oil-free or powder-based makeup as desired.

Midday Touchup

1. Keep "crinkle stick" in your bag and when you repair your makeup pat stick gently over any wrinkled area (right over makeup). . .around the eyes, mouth, etc.
2. With dry tissue, blot excess oil and/*or* grime from face. (If you don't wear a foundation, blot oily areas lightly with pads or tissues moistened with skin freshener.)

Evening Routine

1. Apply cleansing cream over entire face. Gently but firmly remove makeup with several clean tissues.
2. Lay several applications of warm, wet washcloth over face to open pores.
3. Apply cleansing cream for a second time and remove with washcloth.
4. Wash face with soap as prescribed in morning routine.
5. Remove any remaining dirt or makeup with skin freshener.
6. Apply eye cream.
*7. Apply protection cream.
8. Blot off excess cream completely.

Once or Twice Weekly Routine

1. Cleanse face as usual with cleansing cream.
2. Wash face as usual with soap.
3. Follow with skin freshener.
4. Steam face for ten minutes.
5. Apply beauty mask of your choice and leave on for amount of time specified in recipe.
6. Remove mask and rinse face thoroughly. Pat dry.

*See notes at end of chapter.

7. Apply skin freshener.
8. Apply eye cream.
*9. Apply protection cream.
10. Blot off any excess cream completely.

Monthly Facial

1. Cleanse face as usual with cleansing cream.
2. Wash face as usual with soap.
3. Follow with skin freshener.
4. Apply protection cream to face. Cover face with wet, warm washcloth and lie down to rest for ten minutes.
5. Remove cream with skin freshener.
6. Steam face for ten minutes. Pat dry.
7. Apply beauty mask of your choice. Place cotton pads soaked in rose water or witch hazel over eyes.
8. Lie down and rest for specified time.
9. Remove mask and rinse face thoroughly. Pat dry.
10. Apply skin freshener.
*11. Apply protection cream.
12. Apply eye cream.
13. Blot off any excess cream completely.

Antiwrinkle Routine for Combination Skin

The most common combination skin is oily in the "T" zone — i.e., forehead, nose, and chin — and either normal or dry in all other areas. The following program is for that combination.

Morning Routine

1. Lay several applications of warm, wet washcloth over face to open pores.

*See notes at end of chapter.

2. Smooth cleansing cream for normal and dry skin over face. Massage well only on normal or dry areas. Remove with washcloth.
3. This step is optional, but if you want to wash with soap and water, now is the time.
4. With short, firm strokes upward and outward, cleanse face with cotton pads moistened with the appropriate skin fresheners (you'll need two lotions). Use fresh cotton as needed and cleanse until pad is free of dirt.
**5. Apply moisturizing cream for normal and dry skin to entire face and massage normal or dry areas deeply.
6. Apply eye cream.
7. Blot off excess cream from normal or dry areas and firmly *wipe off* cream from oily areas with a tissue. (Enough cream will remain to protect the oily areas under makeup or against the weather without adding extra oils.)
8. Spray face lightly with mineral water and let dry naturally.

Midday Touchup

1. Keep "crinkle stick" in your bag and when you repair your makeup pat the stick gently over any wrinkled area (right over makeup). . .around the eyes, mouth, etc.
2. Blot off any excess oil or grime with dry tissue. (If you don't wear a foundation, you can blot oily areas lightly with a pad moistened with skin freshener.)

Evening Routine

1. Apply cleansing cream over entire face. Gently but firmly remove makeup with several clean tissues.

**See notes at end of chapter.

2. Lay several applications of warm, wet washcloth over face to open pores.
3. Apply cleansing cream for a second time and remove with washcloth.
4. Optional wash with soap and water.
5. Remove any remaining dirt or makeup with skin fresheners.
**6. Apply moisturizing cream to entire face and massage normal or dry areas thoroughly.
7. Apply eye cream.
8. Blot off excess cream from normal or dry areas and *wipe* cream off oily areas with a tissue.
9. Spray face lightly with mineral water and let dry naturally.

Weekly Routine

1. Cleanse face as usual with cleansing cream.
2. Optional wash with soap and water.
3. Follow with skin fresheners.
4. Steam face for ten minutes.
5. Prepare only half recipe for a mask for oily skin and half recipe for a mask for normal or dry skin. Apply beauty masks and leave on for amount of time specified in recipes.
6. Remove masks and rinse face thoroughly. Pat dry.
7. Apply skin freshener to oily areas.
**8. Apply moisturizing cream to entire face and massage normal or dry areas deeply.
9. Apply eye cream.
10. Blot off excess cream from normal or dry areas and *wipe* cream off oily areas with a tissue.
11. Spray face lightly with mineral water and let dry normally.

**See notes at end of chapter.

Monthly Facial

1. Cleanse face as usual with cleansing cream.
2. Optional wash with soap and water.
3. Follow the skin fresheners.
4. Apply moisturizing cream to normal or dry areas only. Massage thoroughly.
5. Cover face with warm, wet washcloth and lie down to rest for ten minutes *or* steam face for ten minutes.
6. Remove cream with skin freshener.
7. Apply appropriate beauty mask to each skin type area. Place cotton pads soaked in rose water or witch hazel over eyes.
8. Lie down and rest for specified time.
9. Remove masks and rinse face thoroughly. Pat dry.
10. Apply skin fresheners to oily areas.
**11. Apply moisturizing cream to entire face and massage normal or dry areas deeply.
12. Apply eye cream.
13. Blot off excess cream from normal or dry areas and *wipe* cream off oily areas with a tissue.
14. Spray face lightly with mineral water and let dry naturally.

Quickie Facial for Special Occasions — for all Types of Skin

1. Apply cleansing cream and remove as usual.
2. Optional wash with soap and water.
3. Follow with skin freshener.
4. Steam face mildly.
5. Apply moisturizing (or protection) cream as usual.
6. Cover face with warm, wet towel, place pads soaked in rose water over eyes, and lie down for ten minutes.

**See notes at end of chapter.

7. Apply eye cream.
8. Blot off excess cream.
9. Spray face lightly with rose water and let dry naturally.
10. Apply makeup as desired.
11. Have fun.

Footnotes

*If your skin is excessively oily, use the protection cream only when you are intending to apply makeup or to subject your skin to the dirt and grime of outdoor air. If you are going to remain in the house or go to bed, try leaving the skin free of any cream except eye cream. Your natural oils may be enough to keep the skin lubricated. If not, apply a protection cream every time you cleanse your skin.

**If the oily areas are excessively oily, use moisturizing cream on those areas only when you are intending to apply makeup or to subject your skin to the dirt and grime of outdoor weather. If you are going to remain in the house or go to bed, try leaving the oily areas free of any cream. Always be sure to apply moisturizing cream to normal or dry areas. (Another alternative is to make up a batch of protection cream for oily skins and use that on the oily areas.)

6

Face-Saving Formulas

The perception of the beautiful is gradual,
and not a lightning revelation; it requires
not only time, but some study.
                                    —Giovanni Ruffini

A normal, healthy face skin requires regular attention, but a *problem* skin — like a problem child — demands attention *plus* patience and tender loving care. Also, like a child, it demands discipline. . .from without and within.

Let me state at the outset that this chapter is devoted to the care of "troubled" skin. *Unhealthy*, *not* pathological, skin. In view of the multiplicity of causes in such conditions as acne, it would be unwise for me (or you) to diagnose the reason for any persistent eruptions on the face. That is the province of the medical profession.

This book deals with fundamentally normal skin and, although this chapter specifically directs attention to skin that exhibits a degree of abnormality, no attempt will be made to diagnose or prescribe treatment for pathological conditions.

If eruptions are profuse and disturbances long-lived, get advice from a competent dermatologist. Only a doctor is qualified to judge the *cause* of a serious condition and then be able to prescribe a cure.

As for nonserious, but surely disturbing, conditions, the information offered here should be helpful. If you experience merely an occasional breakout, you'll find suggestions which should clear up any blemishes within a short amount of time. If you are experiencing an ongoing series or cycle of pimples, you may have to examine and reevaluate your entire life style.

If you're a teen-ager and have troubled skin, you know you're not alone. The years of adolescence are commonly riddled with skin problems. The body is undergoing physiological changes at an accelerated rate, emotional tensions are often high, and diet is apt to be high in starches and fats if predictable at all.

Whatever your age, the manifestation of eruptions on the skin is a sign of some sort of disorder within the system. It can be as simple as the normal hyperactivity of the sebaceous glands during menstruation. As I mentioned in Chapter One, the output of your oil wells rises perceptibly during that period. It reaches a steady, high level about the twelfth to fifteenth day of the menstrual cycle and maintains that level until the onset of menstruation.

Another possible cause of excessive pimples is the effect an inadequate diet can have on the skin. Many bacteria that lodge quite peaceably within the body when the sugar content is normal raise havoc with the skin when the sugar level is high. If you thrive on starchy foods, gooey desserts, candy, etc., simply cutting those foods out of your diet may terminate your skin problems abruptly. As a general rule, stay away from foods containing starch and sugar. . .such as bread, pastas, waffles, pancakes, potatoes, cakes, pies, cookies, and all sweets and candies.

Oils are another major cause of skin disorders. Pores are not often clogged from without. The grease content of the pores comes from natural changes within the skin, or in the sebum. If the output of the sebaceous glands is heavy, and the oil becomes infected or trapped while seeking its way to the surface, the system will oxidize it and force it to the surface in the hardened form of a blackhead or blemish.

In fact it's necessary to do everything possible to encourage the infected oils to the surface. When germs penetrate the sebaceous glands, the diseased oil becomes contagious and can spread from one oil gland to another. Only deep, deep and thorough cleansing can prevent or minimize this.

To return to diet for a moment, the foods you take into your body can regulate the activity of the sebaceous glands to a great extent. Eliminating fried or greasy foods, oily nuts, rich salad dressings, fatty meats and spicy dishes can help calm your oil glands and clear up complexion problems.

A good nutritious diet of fruits, fresh and cooked vegetables, lean meats, broiled fish and poultry, fresh dairy products, and lots of water will probably help not only your face but your figure and general health as well. There seems to be an impressive amount of evidence to indicate that lack of sufficient vitamins, notably A, D, and B — and to some extent vitamin C — can complicate skin problems. If you suspect a vitamin deficiency in your own diet, you may want to supplement your intake with a good multiple vitamin daily.

Most often, eruptions are caused by the simple fact that the hygiene of the skin is not adequate. That's why *deep cleansing* is emphasized in every chapter of this book. If the normal, healthy functions of the skin are inhibited — by dirt particles, leftover makeup, unexcreted oils, or infectious bacteria (which are supported by the other three) — then a clear complexion is impossible. The skin needs constant care. And it needs it on a long-term basis, not only at the time of a flareup.

Exercise is important, too. Body organs need movement, activity, in order to function properly, and the skin organ is no exception. Your skin will never glow with *life* unless your whole body is awake and alive.

Lastly, in the consideration of skin abnormalities, emotional stress must be mentioned. The face is the outward and visible sign of inward and invisible beauty. . . *or* strain. If you or your dermatologist can fathom no organic causes for skin disorders — and they are chronic and persistent — it's possible you're seeing the wrong kind of doctor. Skin problems can be psychosomatic in origin, and it might be advisable to consult a reputable, competent psychiatrist.

All right. So much for the possible causes of troubled skin. What can you do for the *symptoms*, i.e., pimples, while your setting about to correct the cause? The answer is over and over again, *cleanliness and care.* If you are plagued with eruptions, blemishes, boils, pimples — call them what you like — your immediate problem is to clear up the breakouts that are impairing your beauty. In the last analysis, the cure may come from treating something *internally* — either physical or mental — but if you determinedly follow a routine of *deep cleansing* and care of your skin, you can at least help to control the external manifestations.

The program is as follows: First, read Chapter One carefully so you know about the skin's nature and requirements in general. Then, at least twice a day (more often if you can), upon rising and before bed, cleanse the face with a non-penetrating cleansing cream to remove dirt and grime and makeup (if you're wearing it, which I hope you aren't). Next, a thorough soap and water wash. The very reason soap may not be good for other skin types is the reason it's good for yours. Most soaps have a drying effect. Choose a pure, mild, or medicated soap, *rinse well*, and follow the wash with an astringent skin freshener. Finish with the application of a lotion which will act as a skin-drying agent.

If you must apply makeup, choose a medicated product which will help dry the troubled areas while it covers.

It would be better to leave the face free of anything save the drying agents. If the pores are smothered by makeup, they can't breathe and the infection is kept buried. Every effort must be made to allow the skin to function properly and bring the infection to the surface for elimination.

Even before you think of healing, however, the skin must be clean.

Cleansing Creams for Troubled Skin

First open the pores by laying several applications of warm, wet washcloth over the face. Then smooth cleansing cream over face and remove gently with the washcloth. Use a fresh cloth every day to avoid spreading any infection that might cling to it.

APPLYING CLEANSING CREAM

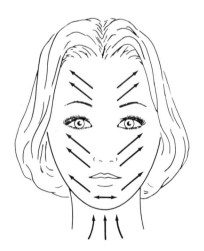

Recipes for Cleansing Creams for Troubled Skin

Creme de Menthe Cleansing Cream

2   tbsp beeswax
3   tbsp petroleum jelly

3 oz mineral oil
2 tbsp witch hazel
2 tbsp creme de menthe extract
1/8 tsp borax

Melt beeswax and petroleum jelly. Warm oil and beat into wax mixture. Dissolve borax in slightly warmed witch hazel and extract. Pour slowly into first mixture, beating constantly. Beat until cool and creamy.

Herbal Cleansing Cream

1 tsp each sage, thyme, oregano
1 cup water
4 tsp beeswax
4 tsp spermaceti
2 oz mineral oil
2 tbsp herb water
1/8 tsp borax

Boil the cup of water and steep herbs in it for two hours. Strain and set aside 2 tbsp of herb water which you will use for the cream. (You can use the rest for a nice steam soup.) Melt beeswax and spermaceti over low heat. Warm mineral oil and beat into wax mixture. Dissolve borax in the 2 tbsp of warm herb water and pour slowly, beating constantly, into first mixture. Beat until cool and creamy. Makes 4 oz.

Medicated Cleansing Cream

3 tbsp petroleum jelly
1 tsp spermaceti
1 1/2 oz mineral oil
2 tbsp grated medicated soap
1 oz rose water
1 tbsp glycerin
1/8 tsp borax

Melt petroleum jelly, soap, and spermaceti over low heat. (Don't worry if the soap doesn't melt completely. It will blend when you mix it.) Warm mineral oil and glycerin together. Beat into first mixture. Dissolve borax in warm rose water and, pouring slowly, beat into mixture until cool and creamy. When using, wash face with warm water using the cream in place of soap. Makes 4 oz.

Carotene Cleansing Cream

      3   tsp beeswax
      2   oz mineral oil
      1   tbsp witch hazel
      1   tbsp fresh, strained carrot juice
    1/8   tsp borax

Melt beeswax over low heat. Warm mineral oil and beat into wax. Heat carrot juice until just below boiling. Add witch hazel and dissolve borax in the warm mixture. Beat, pouring very slowly, into the wax and oil mixture until creamy and cool. Makes 4 oz. Refrigerate.

Petro-Gel Cleansing Cream

1 jar petroleum jelly

That's all. Use as you would any fancy cream.

Simple Liquid Cleanser

1 bottle light mineral oil

That's all. Use as usual.

Skin Fresheners for Troubled Skin

Remember when you're applying a skin freshener that you're not putting lotion *on* your face, you're swiping every last trace of oils, dirt, and grime *off* your face. Moisten a cotton pad with the lotion and then, with upward and outward strokes, wipe the face with gentle, but firm movements. Use several pieces of cotton. Especially with troubled skin, you need to avoid spreading infection, so use a fresh pad for each area. A skin freshener is an all-important beauty aid for you because it removes excess oil and acts as a gentle drying agent at the same time. Use it liberally and often throughout the day.

APPLYING SKIN FRESHENER

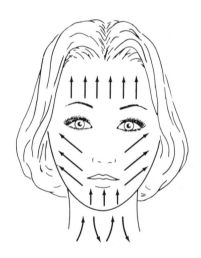

Recipes for Skin Fresheners for Troubled Skin

Peppermint Freshener

1	tsp alcohol
2	oz witch hazel
1	tsp glycerin
1/8	tsp menthol
3	oz alcohol
1/8	tsp tragacanth

Moisten tragacanth with 1 tsp alcohol. Add the witch hazel and glycerin. Dissolve the menthol in the remaining alcohol and add to the first solution.

Apple Freshener

1   oz apple vinegar
2   oz witch hazel
2   oz alcohol

Shake together in bottle.

Rose Water Freshener

1/8   tsp alum
tiny pinch menthol
tiny pinch camphor
1/2   tsp boric acid
1   tbsp alcohol
1   tsp glycerin
2   oz rose water

Filter into bottle through cheesecloth after three days.

Cucumber Freshener

1/8   tsp tincture of benzoin
1/8   tsp alum
1   tsp glycerin
2   oz alcohol
2   oz witch hazel
2   oz cucumber juice

Squeeze or blend one cucumber (skin and all) and strain. Shake all ingredients together in bottle. Very perishable, but very nice! Refrigerate.

Carotene Freshener

3   oz witch hazel
3   oz alcohol
2   oz fresh, strained carrot juice

Shake together in bottle.   Shake before each use. Refrigerate.

Lemon or Grapefruit Freshener

2   oz witch hazel
2   oz alcohol
1/8   tsp alum
1/8   tsp tincture of benzoin
1   oz fresh lemon or grapefruit juice
1   tbsp lemon extract

Squeeze lemon or grapefruit and strain.   Shake all ingredients together in bottle.

Drying Agents

These are a most important health aid for troubled skins as they help to dry and eventually eliminate the blemish itself.   After your face is immaculately clean, dip a cotton swab into one of the following solutions and cover (don't smother!) the pimple.   Each time you wish to reapply the drying agent, cleanse the face afresh with a cotton pad and skin freshener first.

It's impractical to make these lotions up yourself. Any druggist has them on hand and according to the pharmacists with whom I have talked, the following three are the most recommended by dermatologists.

Lotio Alba — this formula is known to almost any druggist and if he doesn't have it already made up, he can mix it together for you in a couple of minutes.

Calamine Lotion — don't agree to any suggestions of adding a small percentage of phenol. It's very potent and can be extremely dangerous if used indiscriminately. Apply the lotion straight.

Liquimat — this comes in light, medium, and dark shades so you can also use it as a coverup.

Fostril or Fastex — this can also be used as a coverup as it is flesh-colored.

Coverups for Troubled Skin

It's much healthier for a troubled skin to go naked (with just a drying agent to aid healing). However, there are times when you want to cover eruptions and the following recipes will allow you to do so, without subjecting your skin to the impurities of makeup.

Neutracolor Coverup

    4   tbsp pure cornstarch
tiny pinch neutracolor
    1   tbsp witch hazel
    1   tbsp camphor water

Mash powders and witch hazel with a mortar and pestle. When a smooth paste, add camphor water and put in small jar.

Benzoin Coverup

    4   tbsp fuller's earth
    2   tbsp rose water
  1/2   tsp tincture of benzoin

Mix rose water into talcum to form a paste. Blend in enough tincture of benzoin to get desired shade. When you put this in a jar, it will harden. Wet finger and rub for each application.

Your Own Foundation Coverup

1 bottle medicated foundation (no rosy shades)
calamine lotion

Pour one-third to one-half of the foundation out. Fill bottle with calamine lotion and shake.

Beauty Masks for Troubled Skins

The application of a facial mask is especially beneficial to problem skins. You receive all of the advantages that a normal skin receives, but they *mean more* to an abnormal skin. Because your skin is irritated, the softening action of a good mask imparts a more than just welcome smooth look. Masks that tighten and minimize pores refine the appearance of the skin and also provide an additional drying effect. And more than anything else, a mask stimulates circulation which causes internal cleansing. A problem skin must not be massaged because that would excite the sebaceous glands and encourage them to produce more oil, which is exactly what you don't need. But beauty masks can draw the blood to the surface which will feed the tissues *and* take along with it on its return trip many of the impurities which are causing trouble on the surface.

Certain masks can also pull the infection to the surface so it can be emptied from the pores and allow the pores to breathe normally again.

It's very helpful to apply a beauty mask at least twice or three times a week to afford your skin the really deep cleansing it so desperately needs.

Before applying the mask, it would be a good idea to steam your face. The hydrating warmth opens the pores, unclogs them, and encourages toxins and infected oils to the surface for elimination. It's yet another method of deep cleansing that troubled skin cries for.

If you have a vaporizer (and there are some manufactured especially for this purpose), simply add your homemade soup in the prescribed amount and steam away (unless, of course, your vaporizer specifies the use of plain water only.) If you're sans modern contraption, do it the way grandma did. Heat the soup in a pot; remove from heat and cover your head (and the entire opening of the vessel) with a towel to keep the steam in. It's easy either way.

After a good ten-minute steam, pat your face dry and immediately apply the beauty mask which you have prepared in advance. *Do not apply masks to eye area.*

For both the soups and the masks, I've enumerated the essential properties of each ingredient so you can mix, match, or substitute for them in the recipes.

Always apply a beauty mask to a clean face. Let me warn you that masks are messy, so wear either nothing at all from the waist up or something old covered with a towel to catch any drippings. Don't be alarmed. You'll get used to it, and when you see the great results I don't think you'll mind. Masks may be a mess, but for troubled skin they're definitely a must. . .so you might as well have some fun with them.

Recipes for Steam Soups

Sage Soup (astringent, pore opener)

Place a handful of dried sage leaves in 1 qt of boiling water. Let steep for a couple of hours. Bring to boil again, remove from heat, and steam face for ten minutes. Leftover soup can be stored in refrigerator and reused.

Thyme Soup (astringent, pore opener)

Use either fresh or dried thyme and follow Sage Soup recipe.

Mint Soup (astringent, pore opener)

Use either fresh or dried mint leaves and follow Sage Soup recipe.

Recipes for Beauty Masks for Troubled Skin

(You can also use any of the beauty mask recipes for *oily skin* in Chapter Six)

Peppermint Pack

3-4 tbsp wheat germ (protein)
1   tbsp peppermint extract (pulling power)
1   tbsp water

Blend extract and water into wheat germ to form a spreadable paste. Apply to face and let remain for fifteen minutes. Remove with warm water and follow with a splash of cold. Pat face dry.

Egg White Mask

1   tsp camphor oil (drying qualities)
1   egg white (pulling power, tightening)

Whip slightly and apply to face. When first layer is dry, add a second and then a third layer. Let remain on face for fifteen minutes and remove with warm water followed with a splash of cold.

Carrot-Clay Pack

1   oz carrot juice (astringent, vitamin A)
2   oz fuller's earth (pulling power, drying qualitites)
2   tbsp tincture of benzoin (antiseptic)

Add tincture of benzoin to fuller's earth and work in enough carrot juice to form a soft clay. Apply to face and let remain for twenty minutes. Remove with warm water followed with cold.

Bran 'n' Buttermilk Mask

3   tbsp pulverized bran (skin softener)
4   tbsp buttermilk (skin softener, bleach)

Pulverize bran in blender or mash until fine. Blend in buttermilk to form a soft paste and apply to face. Leave this soothing, softening mask on for twenty minutes and remove with warm water. Splash with cool water and pat dry.

Almond-Oat Scrub

3   tbsp pulverized oatmeal (protein, abrasive vehicle for soap and water mix)
1   tbsp shaved castile or medicated soap (drying agent)
1   tbsp water
1   tbsp almond extract (scent)

Pulverize oatmeal in blender or mash fine. Add soap and pour water into mixture, mixing well, a little at a time, until a spreadable paste is formed. Blend in almond extract. Apply to face and let remain for twenty minutes. When removing with warm water, use a gentle washing motion to benefit from the slight abrasive action of the oatmeal. (Do not use if you have open wounds). Follow with cool rinse.

Herb-Protein Mask

1   egg yolk (protein)
1 1/2 tsp dried sage (astringent)
1 1/2 tsp dried mint (astringent, pulling power)
1 1/2 tsp dried thyme (astringent)

Whip the yolk until pale yellow and thick. Mix in herbs and apply to face. Let remain for twenty minutes and remove with warm water.

AfterMask

After removing the mask, check your face carefully for black- or whiteheads that are ready to be pressed out from the pores. *Caution must be taken when emptying clogged pores.* Take a tissue and tear it in half. Cover both index fingers and press gently, but firmly, on either side of the blemish. Only remove that infection which dislodges without effort. *Do not apply great pressure.* Re-cover the fingers with a clean section of the tissue for each separate removal. *Be careful that you don't spread the infection.* Use fresh tissues as necessary. (Do not squeeze any sort of blemish on the nose. If done improperly and infection ensues, it can drain directly to the brain and prove fatal. If you have persistent bumps on the nose, see a dermatologist.)

When the face is clean, wipe it gently with a cotton pad moistened with the skin freshener of your choice to disinfect the area. Let the face dry naturally and then cover (don't smother!) blemishes with a drying agent.

Beauty Routines for Troubled Skin

Now that you know how to prepare and use all of the separate concoctions, I think it might be helpful to outline some regular beauty routines.

Once you get into the habit, it won't require more than a few extra minutes a day, and the results should be well worth it. The important thing is to establish the habit.

Daily, weekly, and monthly routines follow.

Morning Routine

1. Lay several applications of warm, wet washcloth over face to open pores.
2. Smooth cleansing cream over face. Remove with washcloth.
3. With pure or medicated soap, wash face thoroughly. Rinse well — many *times* — splashing warm then cool water repeatedly over face. Pat dry.
4. With short, firm strokes upward and outward, cleanse entire face with cotton pads moistened with skin freshener. Use fresh cotton as needed and cleanse until pad is free of dirt.
5. Apply drying agent or covering lotion.
6. Apply eye cream (see Chapter Five).
7. Apply any eye or other makeup as long as makeup does not come into contact with eruptions.

Midday Touchup

1. Keep "crinkle stick" in your bag and, when you repair your makeup, pat stick gently over any wrinkled area around the eyes, mouth, etc.
2. Blot erupted areas with pads moistened in skin freshener, let dry naturally, and re-cover with drying agent or cover lotion.

Evening Routine

1. Apply cleansing cream over entire face. Gently, but firmly, cleanse face with several clean tissues.
2. Lay several applications of warm, wet washcloth over face to open pores.
3. Wash face with soap as prescribed in morning routine.
4. Wash face a second time with soap and water.
5. Finish cleansing with cotton pads moistened in skin freshener.

6. Apply drying agent to erupted areas.
7. Apply eye cream.

Twice or Thrice Weekly Routine

1. Cleanse face as usual with cleansing cream.
2. Wash face as usual with soap.
3. Follow with skin freshener.
4. Steam face for ten minutes.
5. Apply beauty mask of your choice and leave on for amount of time specified in recipe.
6. Remove mask and rinse face thoroughly. Pat dry.
7. Remove blackheads. (Once a week.)
8. Apply skin freshener.
9. Apply drying agent to erupted areas.
10. Apply eye cream.

Monthly Facial

1. Cleanse face as usual with cleansing cream.
2. Wash face as usual with soap.
3. Follow with skin freshener.
4. Steam face for ten minutes.
5. Apply beauty mask of your choice and leave on for amount of time specified in recipe.
6. Remove mask and rinse face thoroughly. Pat dry.
7. Remove blackheads.
8. Apply skin freshener.
9. Cut holes for eyes and mouth out of a square of cheesecloth. Saturate cloth with drying agent and cover face. Lie down and rest for ten minutes.
10. Rinse face with tepid water and pat dry.
11. Apply skin freshener.
12. Apply drying agent to erupted area.
13. Apply eye cream.

7

Better Late Than Never

It is never *too* late to improve your appearance by beginning a good skin care program. Even if you are entering or well into your "later" years and see that your skin has begun to show the results of a lifetime of neglect, there is still a great deal you can do not only to restore a more youthful look but also to actually retard outward appearances of the inevitable aging process.

The skin on the face, of course, proclaims the years more nakedly than any other part of the body. And the reason that it does is precisely because of its "nakedness." The face is really the only area which is virtually never covered by some type of clothing — even our hands are protected by gloves in the winter. The best we do for our faces is to occasionally wear a hat to shade it from the sun, but even then, it is exposed to all the other elements of nature, not to mention additional pollutants contributed by man.

Luckily, as long as any damage to the skin is confined to the outer layer, most signs of neglect or aging can be substantially improved. (Read Chapter One thoroughly at this point in order to get acquainted with the skin in general. You will then be better able to understand the particular problems of aging skin.)

108

If any damage has occurred to the dermis, or inner layer, there is really little if anything that can be accomplished with external beauty care. Since the dermis cannot regenerate itself like the outer layer can, any structural damage is usually permanent. Whether the damage has occurred from illness, accident or neglect, the signs will often begin to show with age because it is the dermis which determines the "tone" or elasticity of the skin. It is made up of "bundles" of intertwined elastic fibers which, in time, become dry and brittle and tend to break into little pieces rather like a rubberband which has been lying around too long. Then, with the loss of resilience, the supporting tissues underneath the dermis lose their strength and the whole face begins to sag. Structural collapse, serious wrinkle problems, and scars caused by damage to the dermis are the province of the medical profession. If these are your problems, consult a reputable cosmetic surgeon. It is because of realities like these, of course, that a good preventive skin care program should be followed while you are still young.

However, if the damage has occurred only to the epidermis, or outer layer, the outlook for dramatic improvement is bright indeed. As you read in Chapter One, the outer layer of the skin constantly replaces itself with new cells being produced that work their way to the surface and die there to be sloughed off revealing a nice, new, fresh skin underneath.

One of the problems with aging skin is that it tends to lose its ability to shed the dead skin cells on the surface, leaving them there to build up and give a rough or pasty appearance. That's why it's crucial, at least a couple of times a week, to use a cleansing cream which contains abrasive granules. The little "beauty grains," as we might call them, scrub the dead layer off and leave your face with a younger look immediately.

Another problem common with aging skin is chronic dryness. There are several reasons for this. One is simply the decreased activity of the sebaceous glands — the oil wells are running out of oil and the pumps are not working well either. Another is that, with age, the skin loses its ability to restore the acid balance to the skin if it is altered for any reason; for example, washing with an alkaline soap. Thus a skin freshener is an absolute necessity for aging skin; it replaces the protective acid mantle usually washed away in cleansing. Lastly, the outer cells become less able to hold water, which is, of course, the real moisturizer, and so the skin begins to take on a parched look. The resulting dryness makes even an old skin look older, hence the *need* for a good moisturizing program.

The final insult of aging skin can be a pigment increase in the outer layer. This wouldn't really matter, if it increased evenly, but it tends to do so in a "here and there" pattern which often causes an unattractive splotchy look. This phenomenon is sometimes referred to as "liver spots," but I couldn't tell you why since it has nothing whatsoever to do with the liver. (Some recipes for "liver spot" bleaches will be found in Chapter Ten.)

Obviously, because of these special attributes of aging skin, special care must be given to it. But even if all of your problems seem a little grim, and even if your own face in the mirror shows its age, do not be in the slightest discouraged. *With* special care, it can be dewy and youthful — *lying* its age — within a few short weeks. This chapter is dedicated to making that possible.

Number one: keep your face protected from the elements — from the sun, the wind, and dry heat in particular. Kiss your suntans of yesteryear goodbye and even though you may continue to moderately tan your body, rely on a good face bronzer to fake a tan on your face. *Always* wear a moisturizing cream or oil to help your skin retain its water and at the same time to provide a barrier against exterior toxins and pollutants. And lastly, avoid baking your skin to further dryness by standing over a hot stove, (who wants to do that anyway?) sitting for prolonged periods near a blazing fireplace, (which everybody wants to do) and taking sauna baths. On this last point, treat yourself to a steam bath instead. It will offer you the heat and relaxation you want and, at the same time, surround you with tiny water particles that will prevent your skin from drying out. In the winter, when the artificial heat in your home is drawing moisture from everything it can — from your furniture to your face — keep a humidifier going at all times to replace moisture into the air.

Number two: don't misuse your facial skin. Wear lighter-textured makeup which can't find its way into wrinkles as easily as heavy makeup. Don't wear *anything* in powder form — and that includes *powder*. Powder, powder blushers, and powder eye shadows only dry out and deepen any lines or crevices already on the skin. Stay away from them like the plague! Avoid alkaline soaps if you still wish to use a soap and water wash in your cleansing routine. Try to buy soaps with a pH factor similar to the skin (4.5 − 5.5). Avoid soaps with perfumes or deodorants and lean heavily on some of the newer, superfatted (or moisturizing) soaps. Don't be misled. This latter group doesn't actually *moisturize* the skin, but they are kinder to it because they are less drying. And finally, don't traumatize the skin. Do not use *hot* or *cold* water — just nice, soothing lukewarm, or cool water, when called for.

Number three: encourage the fundamental health of your skin. One of the reasons people look "old" is because they have stopped acting and thinking "young." Inactivity is anathema to the skin, as it is to the entire body. Not only must it, like every other organ of the body, receive the proper nutrients, but it must also *move*.

Without physical activity, the nutrients can't be distributed properly, and the blood (which feeds the skin) never reaches the surface of the skin to deposit its precious oxygen. Even if your lifestyle has become more sedentary, eat properly and get at least moderate exercise. Almost everyone can certainly take long walks and perhaps swim on a regular basis. Yoga, also, is a good form of exercise for practically anybody, of any age, since it requires very little in the way of exertion.

Number four: follow the simple, natural beauty routines in this book. Even if you don't *feel* younger, I believe you will begin to *look* younger. . .which, by the way, has an astounding ability to make you feel younger.

CLEANINGS CREAMS FOR AGING SKIN

First, read Chapter Two of this book in order to understand the principles behind the preparation of creams in general and why certain ingredients are used for certain skin types. You will then understand why all of the creams here are based in penetrating vegetable oils rather than the more (commercially) common mineral oil. Since one of the special problems of aging skin is dryness, you may also select and use any of the recipes in Chapter Two that are designed specifically for *dry* skin.

You should use, however, either the "Oatmeal Cleansing Scrub" or the "Strawberry-Almond Cleansing Scrub," two or three times a week. The little "beauty grains" in each will help remove any dead cell accumulation characteristic of aging skin. You may find it helpful to "wash" your face with these creams using a complexion brush to work the grains around on the surface of your skin. If not, use your fingers or a washcloth. Always remember to scrub *gently*. The grains will do the work for you all by themselves; there is no need to sandpaper your face.

Because the beauty aids in this chapter focus on aging skin in particular, you may be wondering about the use of hormones, which are contained in some commercially-available products. I do not believe in them. Hormones, even when topically applied (as in a cream) change the metabolism of living tissue. It causes it to expand and sort of "plumps" out the skin which can make it look more firm. However, there is considerable controversy in the medical profession over the safety of long-term use of externally applied hormones. The problem is this: hormones cause a *physiological* change in the tissues and thus takes any cream containing them out of the "beauty aid" category, and, in my opinion, puts them into a "medical" category. However, even when recommended by a doctor, I feel the benefits of hormones are insignificant compared to the risks involved.

With all cleansing creams for aging skin, begin by wetting the face with warm water and then apply the cream. You will notice that in all "Antiwrinkle" routines for aging skin, that I constantly combine oil (creams), water, and warmth which help to intensify the moisturizing process which your skin needs.

Recipes for Cleansing Creams for Aging Skin

Crisco Cleansing Cream

That's all. Crisco is merely a combination of hydrogenated vegetable oils and works beautifully as a cleansing cream. It has been used for years by theatre people to remove stage makeup.

Vegetable Cleansing Oil

If you prefer a liquid cleanser, any vegetable oil of your choice will work as well as the fanciest cream. And, if you purchase it in a health food store, you will get an oil totally devoid of any preservatives. You can't get purer than that.

Oatmeal Cleansing Scrub

1   oz cocoa butter
2   oz almond oil
1   oz rose water
1   tbsp beeswax
1/4   tsp borax
2-3   tbsp pulverized oatmeal (not the instant type)

Pulverize oatmeal in blender and set aside. Melt beeswax over *low* heat. Melt cocoa butter separately and add to warm almond oil. Dribble oils into beeswax (off the fire) beating constantly. Warm rose water and borax and beat into mixture until creamy and cool. Beat in oatmeal. Makes 4 oz. Refrigerate.

Strawberry-Almond Cleansing Scrub

1   tbsp beeswax
2   oz peanut oil
1   tbsp strawberry juice
1   tbsp witch hazel
1/4   tsp borax
Pulverized almonds

Liquefy strawberries in juicer or blender. Strain and set aside. Melt beeswax over *low* heat. Warm peanut oil and pouring slowly, beat into wax. Heat 1 tbsp of the strawberry juice with the witch hazel and borax and, pouring slowly, beat into mixture until cool and creamy. Beat in almonds. Makes 3 oz. Refrigerate.

Because of the particular needs of aging skin, these scrubs (which you may vary any way you like, as long as the grains are included) are the only variations necessary beyond what would be offered to you by any other cream designed especially for *dry* skin. Because of this, in addition to these scrubs, you may use any of the other recipes found in Chapter Two under the *dry* skin section.

SKIN FRESHENERS FOR AGING SKIN

Remember when you're applying a skin freshener that you're not putting lotion *on* your face, you're wiping every last trace of oils, dirt, and grime *off* your face. Remember, too, that, especially for aging skin, a skin freshener is restoring the proper acid balance to your skin, hence protecting it.

Moisten a cotton pad with the freshener and then, with upward and outward strokes, wipe your face with gentle, but firm movements. Use several pieces of cotton if necessary until no more dirt is apparent.

Recipes for Skin Fresheners for Aging Skin

Witch Hazel Skin Freshener

That's all. Use as you would any fancy brand. It will work just as well or even possibly better because it is absolutely pure.

Strawberry or Cucumber Skin Freshener

2	oz strained strawberry or cucumber juice
3	oz witch hazel
1	oz alcohol (eliminate if skin is *very* dry)
1	tbsp vegetable oil

Shake all together in bottle. (Refrigerate Cucumber freshener.)

Rose Water Skin Freshener

3	oz rose water
1	oz alcohol
1	tsp vegetable oil

Shake all together in bottle.

Grapefruit, Lemon or Lime Skin Freshener

Fruit of your choice
3   oz alcohol
4   oz witch hazel
1   tbsp vegetable oil

Peel fruit (avoid including white pith with peels) and cut into thin strips. Place alcohol in small glass bowl and add 2 tbsp of the peels. Let stand, covered tightly, for three days. Reserve 2 oz of the flavored alcohol. Add all other ingredients and shake well in bottle. (You may note that in all skin fresheners for other types of skins, the actual juice of these citrus fruits is used. However, these juices are too astringent for an aging skin, and by soaking the peels in this manner, the *oils* of the fruit peel are extracted giving you all of the fruit's refreshing attributes and aroma without its full strength.)

Chamomile Skin Freshener

2   oz chamomile tea
4   oz witch hazel

Shake together in bottle.

Do not use recipes for skin fresheners from the dry skin section of Chapter Two. Your needs are not satisfied by products designed for dry skin alone.

MOISTURIZING CREAMS FOR AGING SKIN

With moisturizing creams, a gentle upward and outward massage should be employed to stimulate circulation of the blood, which will, in turn, nourish the skin. A gentle massage will also stimulate and strengthen the underlying muscle fiber which will help maintain the elasticity of the skin. For specific massage techniques, see the illustrations in Chapter Two under the *dry* skin section. However, do not massage too deeply; a gentle but firm motion is adequate for an aging skin which will no longer benefit from a strong massage.

After you have worked the cream well into your skin, spray some mineral water or rose water (keep it in an old, well-scrubbed Windex bottle) lightly over the face. It will help the cream penetrate and hydrate your thirsty skin at the same time.

Recipes for Moisturizing Creams for Aging Skin

Honey-Rose Moisturizing Cream

2	oz sesame oil (or 1 oz sesame oil and 1 oz rose-scented oil)
1	tbsp beeswax
1	oz rose water
1/4	tsp borax
1	tbsp honey
1	tsp liquid lecithin
2-4	drops red food coloring

Melt beeswax over *low* heat. Warm oil, honey and lecithin together and dribble into wax beating constantly. Warm rose water and borax and, pouring slowly, beat into mixture until cool and creamy. Makes 3 oz. Refrigerate.

Coconut Moisturizing Cream with Vitamins A, D and E

1	oz wheat germ oil
2	tbsp anhydrous lanolin
2	tbsp cocoa butter
1	tbsp coconut oil
1	oz plus 1 tbsp coconut extract
2	tsp liquid lecithin
1/4	tsp borax
10	vitamin pills each vitamin A and D

Melt cocoa butter and coconut oil and add to warmed wheat germ oil, lanolin and lecithin. Beat together thoroughly. Warm extract and borax and, pouring slowly, beat into mixture until cool and creamy. Prick vitamin pills with a pin and squeeze into cream. Beat again until fluffy. Makes 3 oz. Refrigerate.

Blended Oils Moisturizing Liquid

1   oz almond oil
1   oz wheat germ oil
1   oz avocado oil
1   oz coconut oil
1   oz castor oil
1   tbsp liquid lecithin

Heat all together and beat well until thoroughly mixed (don't be concerned if mixture becomes foamy). Cool and put in bottle. Refrigerate.

Vegetable Oil Moisturizing Liquid

Vegetable oil of your choice

Face-Butter Moisturizing Cream

1 container any brand margerine

That's all. Margerine is already a solidified mixture of oils (note soy oil on the package) which works wonderfully as a moisturizer for women who don't care to make their own.

Special Over-Night Moisturizing Cream

1   oz castor oil
1   oz coconut oil
2   tbsp anhydrous lanolin
1   oz wheat germ oil
1   tbsp liquid lecithin

Heat together and beat thoroughly (don't be concerned if mixture becomes foamy). Cool and pour into bottle.

You may also use any of the moisturizing creams listed in Chapter Two under the *dry* skin section, for variety. However, I do not recommend them on a regular basis because the recipes in *this* chapter have been designed especially for an aging skin. When using these recipes, you should not substitute ingredients for I have used certain oils for the properties they alone possess.

BEAUTY MASKS FOR AGING SKIN

Begin by reading the general information on beauty masks — the whys and wherefores — in Chapter Four. All of that applies to an aging skin as well. . .and more. Beauty masks are even more important to an aging skin because of severe dryness and dead-cell buildup. Therefore, your masks are designed to both moisturize and/or remove cells along with the usual benefits of a *deep* internal and external cleansing.

I recommend only one "steam soup," and that is Chamomile Steam soup. These soups are used primarily, of course, to soften the outer layer of the skin and to open the pores so that the subsequent mask application can clean deeply. Chamomile is the mildest, therefore the best for an aging skin. Check Chapter Four under the dry skin section to see how to make and use it. On to beauty masks.

Beauty Masks for Aging Skin

Deep Penetrating Hot Oil Mask

1/2   cup virgin olive oil (moisturizer)
1   square cheesecloth

Cut out a mask from the cheesecloth to fit your face, leaving holes for your eyes and mouth. Warm the olive oil and soak cloth in it. Wring out lightly and fit to face. As cloth cools, dip again into warm oil and reapply. Repeat several times. Rinse oil off your face with warm water and pat dry. A nice, dewy coating will remain to protect you.

Protein Scrub Mask

1   egg yolk (protein)
1   tbsp castor oil (moisturizer)
2   tbsp table salt (abrasive)
1   tsp lemon juice (works with oil to remove dead-cell layer, can be eliminated if skin is sensative)

Mix all together and spread on face. Let remain for twenty minutes. Remove with warm water, but while doing so, use a washing motion (*gently* — salt is *very* abrasive) to benefit from the beauty grains of salt. Splash face with cool water and pat dry.

Honey-Almond Scrub Mask

1/4   cup honey
2   tbsp pulverized almonds

Pulverize almonds in blender and mix into honey. Spread on clean face and leave for twenty minutes. When removing with warm water, be sure to use the washing motion to benefit from the beauty grains of almonds.

Oatmeal-Milk Scrub Mask

1/2   cup milk
Pulverized oatmeal

Pulverize oatmeal in blender (do not use instant type). Add to milk until a thick paste is formed. Spread on face and leave for twenty minutes. Remove with warm water and use a washing motion to gain benefit from the beauty grains of oatmeal. Splash face with cool water and pat dry.

You may also use all of the beauty masks for *dry* skin in Chapter Four. They will prove beneficial to your skin as well. However, be sure to use one of the scrub masks, here in your own chapter, periodically so that you will not accumulate a dead-cell buildup. As you will note in the "Antiwrinkle" section which follows, I recommend the use of a superficial peeler at least once a month as a MUST for an aging skin. You will find recipes for them at the end of Chapter Four.

ANTIWRINKLE ROUTINES FOR AGING SKIN

Now that you understand *why* aging skin requires special care and *how* to make all of your special products, the next step is to determine *when* to apply what you've learned. The important thing is to establish a habit. Granted that hereditary and other previously mentioned factors have played their role in the present condition of an aging skin, but one of the most frequent reasons skin begins to *look* older as it grows older is because good skin care habits were not acquired earlier in life. Better late than never, true, but better today than tomorrow.

You should cleanse your face thoroughly twice a day – in the morning and before bed. In order to care for your skin properly, you should also apply a beauty mask once a week. Then, add to that a monthly facial and you have your entire "antiwrinkle" routine. For aging skins, I also recommend a superficial peeler once a month.

Antiwrinkle Routines for Aging Skin

Morning Routine

1. Wet face with warm water and smooth cleansing cream over face. Massage gently. Place warm, wet washcloth over face two or three times. Remove cream with washcloth, fingers or complexion brush using washing motion if cream contains beauty grains.
2. This step is optional, but if you wish to use a soap and water wash (with a superfatted, pure soap, please) now is the time. Rinse *very* well with warm water and pat dry.
3. With short, firm strokes upward and outward, cleanse entire face with cotton balls moistened in skin freshener. Use fresh cotton as needed and cleanse until pad is free of dirt.
4. Again place warm, wet washcloth over face two or three times. Apply moisturizing cream and massage gently. Place warm, wet washcloth over face one last time.
5. Apply eye cream.
6. Blot off any excess cream.
7. Spray face lightly with mineral or rose water and let dry naturally.
8. Apply oil-based or cream makeup as desired. No powder — it only deepens lines and crevices.

Midday Touchup

1. Keep "crinkle stick" in your bag, and when you repair your makeup, pat the stick gently over any wrinkled area (right over makeup). . .around eyes, mouth, etc. Be sure to smooth out any makeup which may have found its way into crevices.

2. Blot off any grime with a tissue lightly moistened with warm water.

Evening Routine

1. Apply vegetable oil over entire face. Gently but firmly remove makeup with several clean tissues.
2. Apply cleansing cream and remove as in morning routine.
3. Optional wash with soap and water.
4. Remove any remaining dirt or makeup with skin freshener.
5. Place warm, wet washcloth over face two or three times. Apply moisturizing cream and massage face thoroughly. Place warm, wet washcloth over face one more time.
6. Apply eye cream.
7. Blot off any excess cream.
8. Spray face lightly with mineral or rose water and let dry naturally.

Weekly Routine

1. Cleanse face as usual with vegetable oil or cleansing cream.
2. Optional soap and water wash.
3. Follow with skin freshener.
4. Wet face with warm water and apply moisturizing cream and eye cream on wet face.
5. Steam face for five to ten minutes.
6. Remove creams with skin freshener.
7. Apply beauty mask of your choice and leave on for amount of time specified in recipe.
8. Remove mask and rinse face thoroughly. Pat dry.

9. Place warm, wet washcloth over face two or three times.   Apply moisturizing cream and massage thoroughly.
10. Apply eye cream.
11. Blot off any excess cream.
12. Spray face lightly with mineral or rose water and let dry naturally.

Monthly Facial

1. Cleanse face as usual with vegetable oil or cleansing cream.
2. Optional soap and water wash.
3. Follow with skin freshener.
4. Apply eye cream.
5. Wet face with warm water. Apply moisturizing cream to entire (wet) face and throat (including eye area over eye cream). Massage thoroughly.
6. Steam face for five to ten minutes.
7. Remove creams with skin freshener.
8. Wet face with warm water. Apply warm vegetable oil of your choice to entire, wet face and throat.
9. Cover face with warm, wet washcloth and lie down to rest for ten minutes.
10. Remove oil with skin freshener.
11. Apply beauty mask of your choice. Place cotton pads soaked in rose water or witch hazel over eyes.
12. Lie down and rest for specified time for mask.
13. Remove mask and rinse face thoroughly. Pat dry.
14. Apply one of the superficial peelers from Chapter Four. Rinse face thoroughly and pat dry.
15. Wet face with warm water. Apply moisturizing cream over wet face and massage thoroughly.
16. Apply eye cream.
17. Blot off any excess cream.
18. Spray face with mineral or rose water and let dry naturally.

8

There's a Spa in Your Bathroom

. . .I have had a good many more uplifting thoughts, creative and expansive visions — while soaking in comfortable baths or drying myself after bracing showers — in well-equipped American bathrooms than I have ever had in any cathedral.

—Edmund Wilson

My "spa" is four by seven feet, which is about the same small size as many apartment bathrooms. And when I step into this rather intimate spot, my eyes are not drawn to functional white objects, but to others. . .that promise retreat. I am surrounded by flowers that spill from the ceiling to cover the walls. My feet sink into the softness of white sheepskin. Mirrors, fluffs of towels, bottles of homemade oils and scents to anoint. Relaxation awaits.

A bath must always be a beautiful experience. If your only motive is to get clean, then a shower is much more efficient.

And in order to have a beautiful bath, you really ought to have a beautiful bathroom. It's the room most neglected by the most people, even though nearly as much time is spent there as is spent in the living room (so I've heard). The ambience of the living room is created with care, but the average bathroom is considered "done" if it has a colored curtain hung around the shower and a throw rug thrown on the floor. In a New York City bathroom, this decor is often augmented by a box of kitty litter sitting dutifully under the sink. Now, a *spa*, gentle reader, that is *not*.

A beautiful bath *requires* beautiful surroundings. No matter what kind of a bath you have a craving for — a relaxation bath. . .a contemplative or a healing one. . .a bath to read in or sip champagne with a friend in — the room must be well planned.

Richness underfoot is welcoming. Lights that can dim or sconces with candles can soothe the spirit or create romance. Hanging plants that will flourish well in the mistiness can establish an atmosphere of nature so you can "skinny dip" in your own home. Art. Paintings of perhaps flowers and mirrors for real, live nudes. You can pile huge, thirsty towels for afterbath wrapping in inviting view. Devote shiny shelves to beautiful bottles and devote the bottles to clingy scents waiting in homemade oils.

Man has returned to water since the Ancients. . .to heal the body and renew the soul. Create a private sanctuary where you can relax and float free.

Once your personal spa is ready, all you have to do is add the water. *Warm* water. Hot water not only causes the skin to lose some of its elasticity, it's also debilitating and you'll emerge feeling weak and exhausted instead of luxurious and relaxed. Tepid water, on the other hand, will draw the blood gently to the surface to oxygenate the skin and carry away any toxins hiding just under the surface. It will *gently* increase perspiration to help eliminate impurities from the system. And prolonged immersion in such a bath also renders the outer layer of the skin permeable so that many of your fragrant oils can penetrate and soften and smooth every precious inch of your body.

Recipes for Scented Oil Baths

Shower First, Bathe Later Bath

Putting things in this order will give you the fullest possible softening and smelling power from your fragrant bath oil. Leisurely wash your body under the shower, then fill the tub with water. Add bath oil as the water rushes into the tub and slip your nice clean body in to soak. When you're suitably soothed and soft, if bed is your destination, step slowly out of the bath without breaking your relaxed mood, pat yourself dry with the thirstiest towel you can find, and patter off to rest your pampered body. If you're going out, think first of the lovely evening ahead, hop out of the tub, give your body a brisk rubdown to wake it up, and head off for some fun.

Bathe First, Shower Later Bath

As you let the water whoosh into the tub, add the bath oil of your choice. Lie back and float away your cares. When they're all gone away, soap up nice and clean. Your oils will have done their duty before you wash, but this method of bathing leaves you with a drier, less silky feeling afterward. Next, rinse off under the shower as the water runs out of the tub. You may want to use a natural hemp or fiber glove which is excellent for removing dead skin cells. When the last trace of soap has vanished, turn the temperature of the shower water slowly from warm to cool to icy cool. Stimulates circulation and hands you energy at the same time.

Fragrant Oil Shower

It's not necessary to use soap to get clean. Your bath oils (just as your cleansing creams) will do the job just as well and leave you soft, fragrant, and silky besides. Simply let the water run over your body first. Pour a little scented oil onto a wet sponge and wash as usual. Then rinse in warm water followed by cool and then cold. This shower is marvelous for winter, artificial heat-dried skin.

Recipes for Floating Bath Oils

Your Favorite Perfume Bath Oil

4   oz soy oil (do not substitute)
2   tsp your favorite perfume or cologne
1/2 tsp alcohol

Shake gently together in pretty bottle. Add a drop of food coloring for drama and shake before each use. Refrigerate.

Rose Water and Glycerin Bath Oil

2   oz glycerin
1   oz rose water
1   oz light mineral oil
1   tbsp oil of roses (may be omitted)
3   drops red food coloring

Shake together in pretty bottle.

Orange-Almond Bath Oil

2   oz orange extract
2   oz almond oil
1   oz glycerin
1   tsp alcohol
1   drop red and 1 drop yellow food coloring

Shake together in pretty bottle and shake before each use. Refrigerate.

Pine Needle Bath Oil

2   oz pine needle oil
2   oz light mineral oil
1   oz alcohol
1   drop green food coloring

Shake together in pretty bottle and shake before each use. (This lovely oil gives the entire bathroom the woodsy aroma of pines.)

Favorite Flower Bath Oil

1   handful fresh flower petals with a strong aroma from the flower of your choice
1   oz light mineral oil
2   oz glycerin

Let flower petals stand, covered, in a glass bowl with the glycerin for a week or so. Remove flower petals and add the mineral oil and a couple of drops of the food coloring of your choice. Pour the sweet smelling oil into a pretty bottle.

Unscented Glycerin Bath Oil

That's all. This is especially good if you intend slipping into one of your most expensive perfumes after the bath. The glycerin will sleek your body without imparting a scent of its own which would fight the perfume for attention.

Scented or Unscented Moisturizing Bath Oil

Scented: Vegetable oil mixed with scented oils.
Unscented: Plain vegetable oil.
(Also good for after-bath body moisturizer)

Recipes for Healing Baths

Any of the baths in this chapter will help to alleviate a certain amount of emotional stress. However, when you find yourself full of aches or knotted muscles from *physical* activity, one of the following baths should soak away a good deal of the pain.

If your schedule the following day permits, I would suggest that after you slide into one of these baths you then slide right into bed immediately.

Change the linen on your bed so you can crawl between fresh, clean sheets. Turn down the covers and have a comfortable gown laid out. Or let your body rest free of any wrapping except the sheet. Leave one light (low) waiting in the bedroom.

Then with just the glow from a small light or candle, sink into your healing bath. Isolate and relax each part of your body separately. Lean your head against a rubber pillow or a towel rolled up at one end of the tub. Rest. Your muscles and your mind.

Don't shower afterward. Pat yourself dry, blow out the candle, and go *directly* to bed. Sleep until you wake up naturally the next morning. Try not to use an artificial device to wake you up. You have an inner alarm that will let you know when your body is rested.

Healing Bath Recipes

Herbal Bath

2   tbsp each of parsley, sage, rosemary and thyme
1   qt boiling water

Steep herbs in water for two hours. Strain and pour entire quart of herb "tea" into running bath water.

Sea Water Bath

few handfuls sea salt

Keep the salt in a pretty bottle and just add to bath water as desired. If you have a home whirlpool — which is superb for body aches — you can even have waves and pretend you're paying twenty dollars a treatment at some seashore spa.

Epsom Salts Bath

Measure Epsom salts into whichever bottle you intend to use. Pour salts out into large bowl. Add food coloring of your choice. Keep adding color and stirring until desired hue is achieved. Or divide the salts and make three different colors. Then when you put the salts back into the bottle you can have colored layers, or mix them all together like confetti.

If you would like a fragrance, add perfume. Be sure your colored salts are dry and then return them to the bottle.

For bathing, add a few handfuls under the rushing water as it fills the tub.

Wintergreen Muscle Soothing Bath

1   oz methyl salicylate (oil of wintergreen)
1   oz light mineral oil
2   drops green food coloring

Shake together and shake before each use. (1 tbsp is enough to add to your bath; its scent is heavenly, but heady.) DO NOT GET WATER ON FACE. KEEP AWAY FROM CHILDREN. Methyl salicylate really does wonders for aching muscles, but it is a poison, so normal caution is in order.

Sunburn Bath #1

baking soda

That's all. Just add a few handfuls to lukewarm (not even tepid) water and let it take the fire out of your burned body. (And make a sunscreen from Chapter Ten before you go into the sun next time.)

Sunburn Bath #2

tea (choose 6 or 8 bags of strong, black tea)

Tie tea bags together and add them to a *hot* bath. By the time the water cools to lukewarm and is ready for you to step in, your tannic acid "tea" will be ready to soothe the burn.

Recipes for Other Baths

Milk Bath

1   packet powdered skim milk
1   qt cold water
1   oz flavored extract of your choice (optional, but almond & lemon are delicious)

This famous bath will not only whiten your skin but make it feel positively velvety as well. Simply make up the quart of milk, add the scent (or not), and pour the whole thing into your bath and *you* have it as good as Cleopatra. It turns the water pale blue with a heavenly white foam.

Quickie Milk Bath

Just buy powdered milk packets or pour loose powdered milk from the box into a pretty bottle to keep on the shelf. Open a packet or two (or throw a handful or two) into the tub as it fills with water. Voila! A milk bath.

Bubble Bath #1

Shave castile soap with a cheese grater and keep the soap in a pretty box. Add a handful or two under hot, running water. No need to soap up with this bath. You'll soak clean.

Bubble Bath #2

Any nondetergent liquid you would use to wash fine lingerie. Pour a few capfuls under hot, running water.

Recipes for Bath Parties

Now that you have created a secret spa and conjured up some secret recipes, why not share your secrets? I'm not recommending you have a block party in your bathroom, but it can be a lovely thing to invite the man in your life to share your beautiful bath.

If the mood is tender, your bath is an unrivaled place for soft conversation. You can exchange ideas and back rubs at the same time. Serve cool wine or favorite drinks along with elegant canapes.

Keep a jar of macadamia nuts in the medicine cabinet and if the "double dip" is spontaneous surprise him with their hiding place and eat them right out of the jar accompanied by an icy pitcher of martinis.

If you're both feeling feisty and full of fun, have a water fight and play other water games. Use bubble bath instead of scented oils and offer him fruit and cheese with some chilly champagne.

Some recipes for both bathing and eating delights follow to, I hope, entice your imagination. But you can dream up better parties for your special man that I can. . . parties that are personal moments from you to him. Bathing together can be a close, loving experience and it can often lead to other close, loving experiences.

Saturday Afternoon Splash

For all parties, set a small, low snack table near the tub. This is not the time to ask your guest to hold his food in his lap.

Lemon Bath Oil

3   oz lemon extract
4   oz sesame oil
1   drop yellow food coloring

Shake together in pretty bottle. You can add a real lemon peel for drama. Refrigerate.

Sangria (Don't pour in bath. This is to drink!)

1   bottle dry red burgundy
2   oz brandy
2   oz cointreau
1   large orange
1   large lemon
little club soda

Peel orange in one long spiral strip. Set strip aside. Slice orange and place in large, clear pitcher. Peel and slice lemon and add to orange. With a large, *wooden* spoon, press fruit against pitcher to extract as much juice as possible without smashing it. Add one tray of ice cubes. Pour bottle of red wine over ice and fruit. Add brandy and cointreau (more or less cointreau depending upon how sweet you want the drink). Top with a little soda.

Stir with wooden spoon, leave spoon in pitcher, and drape the long orange spiral over the edge of the pitcher so most of it dunks into the wine.

Hold spoon over lip of pitcher each time you pour Sangria into chilled wine glasses so that fruit and ice don't splash into the glass as well. Add one piece of fruit to each glass. When wine is finished, eat fruit which is by this time soaked through with wine.

Saturday Evening Serenade

Oriental Bath Oil

1   tsp oil of musk or
1   tbsp musk scented perfume (add more if you like a stronger
     fragrance)
1 1/2 oz light mineral oil
3   oz safflower oil

Shake together in bottle. Refrigerate.

Pate Verderi pour le Bain

1/2   lb ground calves' liver
1/2   lb ground pork liver
1/2   lb ground pork meat
1/2   lb ground veal
1   large onion (finely chopped)
1/2   garlic bulb (finely chopped)
1/4   tsp each:
         cinnamon
         thyme
         ginger
         tarragon
         oregano
         basil
         nutmeg
salt and pepper to taste

Mix all together. Add 4 eggs. Mix thoroughly with
hands. Butter a mold and fill with mixture. Cover with
thin film of olive oil. Lay 1 bay leaf on top. Bake in oven
at 350° for one-half to three-quarters of an hour. Test
with knife. Pate is done when knife comes out clean.

Finger Shrimps

1 lb unshelled shrimp (jumbo if possible)

Boil 1 quart water in pot.   Add shrimp.   Drain after three minutes and run under cold water.   Can be eaten either chilled or warm.   Serve shrimp with shells still on (part of the fun is unshelling them at the party) in a bowl centered with a smaller bowl of sauce.

Shrimp Sauce

Ketchup with horseradish to taste.

Champagne in a Bucket

Serve in chilled, tulip-shaped champagne glasses, or, if you're reluctant to use your good crystal in the bathtub, plastic champagne and wine glasses are available at most party stores.

Play soft music in the background (don't have an electric radio in the bathroom near water or touch it when wet).   Now might be the time to read some poetry aloud. Have Sunday brunch waiting in the fridge.

Sunday Night Special

Spicy Bath Oil

5	sticks cinnamon
20	whole cloves
2	oz safflower oil
2	oz light mineral oil

Break up four cinamon sticks, mash cloves and shake with oils.   Let stand for one week and strain.   Pour spicy oil into a clear bottle and add 1 cinnamon stick for drama. Refrigerate.

Strawberry Slush

1	bottle Moselblumschen wine
1	pt fresh strawberries

Clean and hull strawberries. Place in small punch bowl or clear pitcher. Mash slightly. Add one tray ice cubes and pour wine over all. Serve in chilled, clear cups with a whole strawberry in the bottom.

Cheese Tray

Gourmandaise
French Port Salut
Camembert
Brie

Serve with one loaf French bread and/or basket Melba rounds.

Surprise Party

1 box any mild soap flakes

Cover box with colored paper and decorate with pictures of the two of you, or favorite places you've been together, or his name, or. . .?

Beer and pretzels for treats.

If you would like to further surprise him, you can give him a present of homemade after-shave lotion. Label a pretty, but masculine, bottle (like one of those tiny wine bottles you get on airplanes) with your name and the name of the after-shave which you can make up from the scent you choose.
Example:

Alexandra York
Lemon-Lime After-Shave

Recipe for Your Favorite Scent After-Shave Lotion #1

3   oz witch hazel
3   oz alcohol
1/2-1 tsp glycerin
1   tsp peppermint extract
1-2   oz your favorite scent extract

Shake together in bottle.

Recipe for Your Favorite Scent After-Shave Lotion #2

3   oz witch hazel
3   oz alcohol
1   tsp peppermint extract
1/2-1 oz scented oil of your choice

9

Hair Fare

Beauty draws us with a single hair.
—Alexander Pope

If the face is the setting for our eyes, then the hair is the frame around them both. And it serves the same purpose as the frame of a painting. Although it may possess beauty in its own right, it should encourage interest in and enhance the beauty of the subject which is framed. In order to do that, its color and style must be in harmony with the subject, and needless to say it must in no way divert the attention of the viewer by being in a state of disrepair.

Nothing — living or inanimate — can be cared for successfully unless and until its nature is properly understood, so it's important to learn just exactly what the hair is all about. Then you'll know *what* you're doing and *why* you're doing before you *start* doing.

There are some interesting myths about hair that are quite commonly accepted, and this chapter will attempt to correct some of the more glaring ones. To begin with, there is a prevalent misconception that each individual hair is made up of a series of tubes, one nesting snugly inside the other. Not so.

The anatomy of hair is one not of tubes but of layers. The outer layer is clear and scaly and is called the *cuticle*. The next layer and actually the main bulk of the hair is the *cortex* and is made up of fairly tough fibers that are bound together lengthwise.

The core of the hair shaft is the *medulla*, and many things can be said about the *medulla*. One is that it can, itself, be made up of two or three or four layers. Another is that sometimes it doesn't even have one layer, because sometimes it isn't even there. It's nonexistent. Another is that it doesn't concern us in the least for the purposes of this chapter but deserves to be included in any complete description of the hair.

Around these three main layers, assuming the medulla puts in an appearance, and forming sort of a protective cloak around the entire hair shaft is the *epicuticle*. This is technically the outermost layer of the cuticle and is made up of flat, interlocking cells.

And unlike the medulla, it is of great concern to us in this chapter. The emergence of protein in hair conditioners may not be just a gimmick to get you to buy new products. And the nature of the epicuticle is the reason why.

The epicuticle is cemented onto the main body of the hair shaft by a thin layer of protein. Unfortunately, this protective cloak can be rather easily damaged. Fortunately, it can often be repaired — kind of recemented — by treatment with protein. Ergo: protein conditioners.

An extension of the tube fallacy is the myth that the growing power of each hair is diminished if it has split ends.

HAIR SHAFT

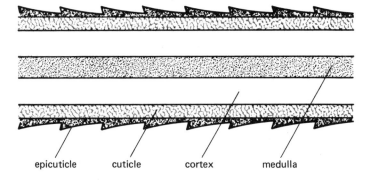

epicuticle   cuticle   cortex   medulla

It is still the custom in Europe, and used to be popular here, to "singe" split ends in order to "close" the "tube" and seal off the ends to promote growth.

What is done to the visible part of your hair may certainly affect the condition and appearance of it, but there is no evidence to indicate that it actually affects growth. Since singeing does eliminate split ends, it isn't necessary to *cut* the hair so often, thus making it *seem* to grow longer, but the growing power of each hair is tucked firmly below the skin's surface.

Each hair shaft has a root which lies beneath the scalp, and that root contains a hair bulb, and it's that hair bulb from which the hair grows. The hair, like the skin, lives out a constant cycle of growing the new and shedding the old. The new, and still actively growing, hair will lengthen somewhere between one half and one inch per month. Once the hair itself is old, no matter how short you cut it or how often you singe it its growing power will terminate, the root will die, and the hair will be sloughed off. As each hair dies, it is replaced (hopefully) by a new one. . .assuming the growing ability remains. If it doesn't baldness is on the way.

Your hair has more growth energy in warm weather than in cold. . .which is the reason why tinted hair needs more touchups in summer than in winter even if it has been protected from the bleaching rays of the sun.

The growing habits of the hair are the reasons, too, why it's a good idea to brush regularly with a natural bristle brush. One hundred strokes a night is *not* a myth. It's a good idea, unless, of course, you have an excessively oily scalp, in which case brushing will cause the oil glands to put out more oil. Besides giving your hair a nice sheen by distributing the oils that accumulate at the base of each hair, it also removes dead hairs which have not yet fallen out by themselves. Better to have them on your brush than on your — or someone else's — shoulder.

A word should be said here about combing the hair. While *brushing* gently removes unwanted hairs, *combing* can pull out or break off healthy hair, so take care. Choose a wide-toothed comb with oval spaces between the teeth. The points of the teeth should be rounded in order to avoid scratching the scalp.

When you're combing *wet* hair, extra caution is necessary. Wet hair loses some of its resistance and can be stretched (which is what curling is) *and* broken more easily. If your hair is wet and tangled, as after a shampoo, start combing gently with short strokes near the ends. Then as that becomes manageable, continue combing, in sections, on up to the base of the crown. With this method, the hairs you see on the comb will be only dead ones; you won't inadvertently have killed some lovely ones just getting started in life. Another note on wet hair. If the weather is warm, try to let your hair dry naturally in the sun. The vitamin D produced by your skin (and that includes your scalp) is healthful, and you also avoid the frequent overdrying effect of a hair dryer.

If you bleach or dye your hair, special babying is required. Unless you are really determined to have one of those pale colors, I would try to convince you to stick to one-process tinting.

The pigment – or natural color – of the hair is contained in the cortex layer. The *natural* color determines the texture. Blonds – very little color – usually have fine hair. On the other end of the spectrum are the redheads with a coarse texture or lots of "body," meaning a heavy cortex layer. Brunettes, depending on the depth of the shade, fall somewhere in between.

Any tinting process is a trauma for hair of any texture. The cuticle has to be softened and opened in order for the chemicals to penetrate the cortex and deposit new color. But with a single process, at least the lightening and coloring processes takes place at almost the same time.

The lightening action works first to open the cuticle and then find its way to the natural pigment in order to lighten it. As soon as the natural pigment has been lightened just enough to receive the new color you've chosen, the coloring action takes over until the hair becomes the desired shade.

A double- or two-process hair coloring is used when you want a drastic change in color. . .drastically lighter, and sometimes drastic for the condition of your hair. If you're a natural brownette and want to become a soft ash or a honey blonde, you can probably do it with a single process. But if you want to go to a champagne blonde a double process would be necessary. "Double process" means that applications of the bleach and color are separate.

The lightener is applied first to "strip" the hair of its natural color. Because it has a lot of lightening to do, it takes a while (usually about an hour) for the bleach to penetrate the cuticle scale and lighten the natural pigment. In some cases, it takes two applications to get the natural color out. After the proper amount of color is removed, turning the hair to straw — that is, straw *yellow* — the new color is put on as a second application. For the next twenty or twenty-five minutes it works its way to the cortex and deposits the pale color in place of the now-removed brown shade. Notice that chemicals are in contact with your scalp and hair at least *three times* as long as with a single process.

Modern hair dyes do a remarkably good job of conditioning the hair while they perform this amazing feat, but with two-step hair coloring, unless the hair is exceptionally sturdy, the results will often be an "unnatural" look ranging from slightly synthetic to cotton candy. Chances are, if your natural hair color is dark, your skin tone won't look well with one of the pastel colors, anyway. I would never advocate that you refrain from changing what Mother Nature gave you, but I really do believe that the fewer unnatural products to come in contact with it the better. And the double process comes close to asking the impossible. No amount of conditioning – natural or unnatural – seems to make hair so harshly treated with chemicals look young and healthy. . .and natural.

Even if you make use of the single process, get to know the treatment section of this chapter. Your hair needs a treatment at least once a week. If you could give yourself one after every shampoo, even better.

And keep your hair clean. As with the skin, cleansing is the single most important issue for the health and beauty of hair – whether it's virgin or violated. Shampoo, preferably with soft water, as often as you feel it's necessary. If you have long hair or a light color or an oily scalp, you'll require frequent shampooing. It's an Old Wives' Tale that lots of washing affects the hair adversely or causes it to fall out. It doesn't do anything except get it clean. . .which is its purpose.

Always follow a shampoo with a rinse. Even if you use a conditioning treatment, pour a rinse through afterward. It will restore the proper pH factor (which is between 4.4 and 5.5 for the hair) and at the same time separate the hairs so each one can individually reflect the light and give your whole head a radiant luster.

Recipes for Shampoos

My best advice on shampoos is to buy them at the dime store. As long as your trusty nitrazine paper (see Chapter One for instructions on what it is and how to use it) indicates that a shampoo is between 4.4 and 5.5, it will probably save you trouble and serve you well. Conditioning treatments and rinses are the products to make at home. In both of these areas you can save a great deal of money and end up with comparable or better products than you could buy. However, if you insist on being a purist, a few tried and true shampoo recipes follow.

When shampooing with any product, if the hair is dry, massage the scalp deeply to stimulate the sebaceous glands. If the hair is oily, merely work the shampoo through the hair completely.

Part Purist Egg Shampoo

At the Five & Ten, select a clear, *cheap* shampoo that checks out to an acidity level of below 7 with nitrazine paper. Break an egg yolk into a plastic cup and beat it until thick and pale yellow. Add 1 ounce of the shampoo and mix well. Shampoo as usual.

Purist Egg Shampoo

This is particularly good for dry or damaged hair as it cleans without removing the natural conditoning effect of your own scalp oils. In addition, it can help to repair the hair with protein.

Beat two or three eggs until fluffy and work them well into hair for at least a full minute. Let them remain for another five to fifteen minutes to benefit from the protein and then rinse out with warmish water. (Not *hot* water or you'll have what might be called an "omelette conditioning cap!")

Old-Fashioned Castile Shampoo

2   oz castile soap
1   qt plus 1 1/2 cup boiling water

Dissolve soap in water and boil slightly. Stir occasionally and add more water if necessary until you have a clear solution. When cool, whip with egg beater until fluffy and scoop a usable amount into a wide-mouthed jar. Store the remaining shampoo in a quart jar. This shampoo will congeal beautifully. All you have to do is dip your fingers into the jar to get enough for a shampoo.

Herbal Shampoo

2   tbsp each:
      parsley
      sage
      rosemary
      thyme
1   qt plus 1/2 cup boiling water
2   oz castile soap

Steep herbs in water for two hours. Strain and follow instructions for Castile Shampoo, substituting herb water. This shampoo leaves a delightful scent to your hair.

Shampoo for Oily Scalp

2   oz castile soap shavings
1   qt plus 1 cup water
3   oz alcohol

Mix soap and water over low heat until dissolved. Whip with egg beater and beat in alcohol. Put usable amount in wide-mouthed jar and store remaining shampoo in quart jar.

Recipes for Hair Treatments

Hot Oil Treatment #1 (for dry or damaged hair)

2-3   oz warm olive oil

Shampoo hair. Towel dry lightly. Section hair and distribute oil near roots. Work through hair thoroughly paying special attention to ends. Wrap entire head with aluminum foil and cover with a shower cap. Sit under hair dryer or heat cap (without the shower cap) for ten minutes. Shampoo hair again and follow with a rinse.

Hot Oil Treatment #2

2-3   oz warm almond oil

Shampoo hair. Towel dry lightly. Heat oil. Pour over hair a little at a time, working the oil well into hair and scalp. With hot curling iron, "curl" small portions (slipping iron the full length) slowly. *Do not touch plug or outlet with wet hands.* Shampoo and follow with a rinse.

Hot Oil Treatment #3

2-3   oz corn oil

Shampoo hair. Towel dry lightly. Heat oil and distribute through hair working in well with fingertips. Wrap hot, steaming towel around head. When towel cools, dip in hot water, wring out, and repeat. Shampoo a second time and follow with a rinse.

Protein Treatment #1

2-3   whole eggs
 1   tbsp lemon juice

Beat the eggs with the lemon juice until fluffy. Work well into wet, clean hair and leave on for twenty minutes. Rinse with barely warm water and follow with the rinse of your choice.

Protein Treatment #2

2-3   egg yolks
1   tbsp apple cider vinegar

Beat egg yolks until thick and pale yellow. Beat in vinegar. (You can use the leftover egg white as a face mask; see Chapter Four.) Work well into wet, clean hair, making sure all hair is covered. Let remain for twenty minutes. Rinse with tepid water followed with a second rinse of your choice.

Mayonnaise Protein Treatment

mayonnaise (any good brand) or homemade mayonnaise

Work through wet, clean hair letting it remain for twenty minutes to one-half hour. Shampoo and follow with the rinse of your choice.

homemade mayonnaise:
2   egg yolks
4   tbsp lemon juice
1 3/4 cups vegetable oil

Beat egg yolks and lemon juice together. Beating constantly, pour a thin stream of oil into the mixture until you have a thick, rich mayonnaise.

Honey Treatment

honey of yor choice

This moisturizes the scalp and slightly bleaches the hair. (But be prepared. It's messy!)
Work into wet, freshly shampooed hair and leave on for twenty-five minutes. Shampoo a second time and follow with the rinse of your choice.

Scented Conditioner

Purchase the pure essential oil of any scent you prefer and brush a *small* amount of it through freshly washed, dry hair to make it manageable, shiny, and fragrant.

Unscented Conditioner

Brush a *small* amount of any vegetable oil *or* glycerin through clean, dry hair to condition it and give it a shiny luster.

Recipes for Rinses

Rosemary Rinse

2   tbsp dried rosemary leaves
1   cup boiling water

Place leaves in water and let steep for two hours. Strain and pour liquid into quart jar filled with three cups warm water. Pour rinse repeatedly through freshly shampooed hair.

Old-Fashioned Vinegar Rinse

1/2   cup white distilled vinegar
1   qt boiling water

Mix, let cool to tepid and pour several times through freshly washed hair. Follow with clear water rinse of coolish water.

Lemon Rinse for Golden Highlights

strained juice of two lemons
1   qt warm water

Mix and pour repeatedly through hair. Follow with clear, warm water rinse.

Lemon Rinse to Slightly Lighten Hair

strained juice of four lemons

Work thoroughly through hair. Sit in the summer sun for fifteen minutes to one-half hour. Rinse hair throughly with clear, warm water.

Chamomile Rinse for Golden Highlights

1   handful chamomile flowers or 6 chamomile tea bags
1   qt boiling water

Let chamomile steep in water until water is tepid. Pour repeatedly over freshly washed hair; let remain for fifteen minutes and rinse with clear, warm water.

Sage Tea Rinse to Darken Hair

1   handful sage leaves
1   qt boiling water

Steep leaves in water for two hours, strain. Pour over hair repeatedly and let remain twenty minutes to one-half hour. Follow with a clear water rinse.

Beer or Champagne Rinse for Extra Body

1 cup any brand beer or champagne

Pour repeatedly through hair. Do not rinse.

Recipes for Wave Sets

Gelatin Set

1   tsp plain gelatin
1   cup boiling water

Mix well. When gelatin dissolves and mixture is cool, comb through hair and set as usual. (Gelatin is also protein, just as an added extra bonus.)

Milk Set

1   tbsp powdered milk
1   cup water

Mix and comb sparingly through hair.   Set as usual.

Beer Set

Comb beer (or dilute it with water for softer look) through hair and set as usual. Or pour beer over hair to wet it and then set as usual. (The smell goes away.)

Wave Set for Normal Hair

5   oz water
1   tsp tragacanth

Soak tragacanth overnight in water. Strain through clean, white cloth. Put in bottle with spray top (an old, well-scrubbed Windex bottle is perfect) and spray onto each section, combing it through as you set hair.

Wave Set for Dry Hair

6   oz water
2   tsp tragacanth
1   tbsp glycerin
1   tbsp plus 2 tsp alcohol
1/8 tsp borax

Mix tragacanth and alcohol in spray bottle. Add other ingredients and shake well. Spray wave set onto each section of hair before setting.

10

Pot of Potpourri

A fair exterior is a silent recommendation.
—Publilius

Once you get to be a beauty cook par excellence, you won't want to spend store prices on *anything* you can make at home.   Be assured; if you can conjure up the idea, you can conjure up the rest in your kitchen.

What comes next is some of the odds and ends *you* may need from time to time and *I* didn't know where else to put.

Some Sun Sense

The sun is not unworthy of being worshipped. It causes the skin to produce vitamin D which is most beneficial to your health. It stimulates the skin to produce a honey-brown glow which is usually beautiful and is called a suntan.

The sun also has a drying effect on the skin. In cases of oily or troubled skins, this can be helpful. The sun gives life, warmth, and light.

The sun is constant and benevolent; it's only our misuse of its nature that can bring us harm. Like anything worthy of worship, it must be respected. Reasonable behavior on our part is in order. Even cautious behavior. Because as well as causing a lovely, lush tan, given enough time the sun can also cause a very painful and not at all lovely burn. And even a moderate sunburn is potentially harmful to the normal function of skin cells. Inflammation caused by a burn can actually damage the cells.

With a little common sense, those very same cells will work *for* you instead of *against* you. Small doses of sunlight will stimulate them to increase a brown pigment called *melanin*. The melanin protects your skin against larger doses of sun and so the cycle is established in your favor. The brown pigment is, of course, the tan we're all after.

Caution — not panic — is desirable too against the drying attributes of the sun. Even if you tan easily and need no protection against the *burning* potential of the sun, you do need protection against its dehydrating potential.

Fortunately, neither burning nor drying the skin is a major problem. Protection against both is achieved simply and inexpensively by the application of an appropriate sunscreen.

Note: A sunscreen doesn't *prevent* the sun's rays from reaching the skin, so exposure must be limited. What a good sunscreen *does* do is absorb a certain percentage of the ultraviolet rays, thus reducing the *intensity* of the sun's powers. This gives your skin a chance to build up its own protection which is the tan you wanted in the first place.

Certain oils absorb more of the ultraviolet rays than others. For this reason, *do not substitute oils* in these recipes. Each has been selected according to its ability to protect your skin.

If a lubricant or sunscreen is *not* used, then the results truly will be a dry, prematurely aged skin. But with the proper care, I can find no facts to substantiate claims that *moderate exposure* to the sun is a danger to any normally functioning skin.

It should be mentioned here too that the facts of the matter also do not support the current, near-hysterical assertions that skin cancer is a threat to average sunbathers. Skin cancer is an occupational hazard of both farmers and sailors, it is true. And it can be caused by the sun. That is also true. But men working in either of these fields are exposed all day, every day, for years on end under the drying effects of the sun. Their skin is seldom if ever protected by even a lubricant, let alone a sunscreen. And with all of this abuse, cases of skin cancer are still rare. I really do not think it looms as a danger for any normal, *reasonable* sunbather.

If you wish to bask in the reflection of that great ball of fire in the sky, I would say to have fun doing it. Just keep firmly tucked away, not too far back in your mind, that fire burns. Don't let it burn you.

Recipes for Sunscreens with Extra Protection for Delicate Skins

Sesame Sunscreen

6   oz sesame oil
1   tbsp oil of bergamot

Shake together in bottle. Keep in refrigerator when not in use.

Coconut Butter Suntan Oil

4   oz sesame oil
2   oz coconut oil
2   oz cocoa butter

Melt cocoa butter and coconut oil over low heat. Warm sesame oil. Stir all together and let cool. Pour into bottle. Refrigerate when not in use. Don't be concerned if it hardens in the bottle. It will melt again at room temperature or in the sun.

Pink Suntan Lotion

1   oz pink calamine powder
2   oz rose water
1   oz sesame oil
1/2 oz glycerin
1   tsp oil of bergamot

Combine in bottle and shake well before each use. Rub well into skin.

Favorite Perfume Sunscreen

6   oz sesame oil
1   tbsp favorite perfume or cologne

Shake together in bottle. Keep in refrigerator when not in use.

Recipes for Complete or Nearly Complete Sunblocks

Zinc Oxide Block

zinc oxide

That's all. Spread on areas where you want total protection from the sun. . .nose, lips, etc. If you want a flesh color, mix with Nutracolor from the drugstore.

Sunblock Cream

2   oz anhydrous lanolin
1   tbsp sesame oil
2   oz rose water
2   tbsp zinc oxide

Melt lanolin and beat in warmed sesame oil. Heat rose water slightly and beat into mixture until coolish. Beat in zinc oxide and put in jar. Refrigerate when not in use.

Wintergreen Sunblock

2   tbsp beeswax
3   oz sesame oil
2   tbsp cocoa butter
1   oz strong, dark tea
1/2   tsp borax
2   tsp methyl salicylate (oil of wintergreen)

Melt, warm, and mix first five ingredients. Beat until cool and add methyl salicylate. Refrigerate when not in use. DO NOT USE NEAR EYES and KEEP AWAY FROM CHILDREN. (Methyl salicylate is a poison, but is commonly used in commercial sunscreens).

Wintergreen Sun Lotion

1   tsp borax
7   oz rose water
1   oz methyl salicylate (oil of wintergreen)
2   tsp glycerin
3   tbsp alcohol

Dissolve borax in water. Add methyl salicylate. Stir until dissolved. Add other ingredients. Shake in bottle and filter through double layer of cheesecloth after a couple of days. Shake before using. DO NOT USE NEAR EYES and KEEP AWAY FROM CHILDREN. (See above note)

Recipes for Sunscreens with Moderate Protection

Peanut Butter Suntan Oil

4   oz peanut oil
2   oz cocoa butter
1   tsp oil of bergamot

Warm oil. Melt cocoa butter over low heat and stir into oil. Cool. Add oil of bergamot and pour into bottle. Refrigerate when not in use.

Sesame Butter Sunscreen

2 oz sesame oil
2 oz cocoa butter
2 oz coconut oil
1 tbsp strong, dark tea

Melt cocoa butter and coconut oil over low heat. Add warmed sesame oil. Beat in warm tea until mixture is cool. Pour into bottle and store in refrigerator when not in use.

Coconut Suntan Oil

4 oz coconut oil
2 oz cottonseed oil
1 tbsp oil of bergamot

Melt coconut oil. Warm cottonseed oil. Stir together. When cool, add oil of bergamot and pour into bottle. Refrigerate when not in use.

Favorite Perfume Suntan Oil

2 oz peanut oil
2 oz sesame oil
2 oz poppyseed oil (coconut oil can be substituted)
1 tbsp favorite perfume

Shake together in bottle and store in refrigerator when not in use.

Olive Sun Oil

4 oz olive oil
2 oz peanut oil
1 oz cottonseed oil
1 tbsp oil of bergamot

Shake together in bottle and store in refrigerator when not in use.

Recipes for Sunscreens with Small Amount of Protection

Coconut Suntan Butter

1 1/2 oz coconut oil
1 1/2 oz cocoa butter

Melt and beat together. Pour into jar and store in refrigerator.   Don't be concerned if it melts in the sun. Refrigerate when not in use.

Favorite Perfume Sun Oil

3   oz mineral oil
3   oz poppyseed oil
1   tbsp favorite perfume or cologne

Shake together in bottle and refrigerate when not in use.

Peanut Butter Suntan Oil

3   oz mineral oil
2   oz peanut oil
1   oz cocoa butter
1   tbsp oil of bergamot

Warm oils. Melt cocoa butter and stir into oil mixture. Let cool, add oil of bergamot, and pour into bottle. Refrigerate when not in use.

Coconut Sun Oil

3   oz coconut oil
3   oz mineral oil
1   tbsp oil of bergamot

Melt coconut oil. Warm mineral oil, stir together, and cool. Add oil of bergamot and pour into bottle. Refrigerate when not in use.

Cocoa Butter Sunscreen

3   oz cocoa butter
2   oz olive oil
1   oz cottonseed oil

Warm oils together. Melt cocoa butter over low heat and stir into oils. Cool, bottle, and refrigerate. Don't be concerned if oil hardens in refrigerator; it will melt again in the sun.

Lubricating Suntan Oils with No Protection

Citrus Suntan Oil

6   oz mineral oil
1   tbsp oil of bergamot

Shake together in bottle.

Cocoa Butter Cream

2   oz cocoa butter
3   oz petroleum jelly

Melt over low heat. Beat until thick. Put in jar and refrigerate when not in use.

Favorite Perfume Sun Lubricant

6   oz heavy mineral oil
1   tbsp favorite perfume or cologne

Shake together in bottle. Shake before each use.

Baby Brown Suntan Oil

6   oz mineral oil
1   tbsp iodine

Shake together in bottle.   Shake before each use.

Recipes for Sunburn Relievers

Recipes follow to help relieve and heal a sunburn should you have failed to read the beginning of this chapter. I hope you'll never have the occasion to prepare one of them. If you do, you might also consult Chapter Seven for some soothing sunburn baths as well.

Touch of Tea Sunburn Lotion

2   oz strong, dark tea
1   tbsp witch hazel
2   oz glycerin

Shake together in bottle and apply to burned areas.

Green Olive Sunburn Helper

2   oz lime water
3   tbsp olive oil
1   tsp borax
1/8 tsp tincture of benzoin

Dissolve borax in lime water and shake in bottle with olive oil. Add tincture of benzoin and shake again. Apply to burn. Shake each time before using.

Vitamin A Sunburn Healer

cod liver oil

That's all. Rub into burned skin; its healing powers are phenomenal.

Massage Oils

I can think of nothing as welcome to a physically fatigued body as a good massage. It can relieve painful, knotted muscles and increase their tone at the same time by stimulating and strengthening the muscle fiber. It circulates the blood and brings it to the surface to nourish and internally cleanse the skin of your entire body. It reduces fat cells. Besides supplementing skin softening oils, it promotes glandular activity within the body. It alleviates stress; nerves are soothed and relaxed. And best of all, it *feels* delicious.

Most masseurs and masseuses use plain mineral oil or a mineral oil-based cream. They are good lubricators and certainly adequate. But I can tell you from many experiences that if you walk in with your own oil your masseuse will love you. The massage oils you can prepare at home offer much better friction and you will get a deeper massage. In addition, they're made with lusciously moisturizing natural vegetable oils which will penetrate your skin and silken your entire body.

Keep all massage oils in the refrigerator when not in use. If they harden or get cloudy, don't be concerned. They will return to their proper consistency at room temperature.

Feel free to substitute oils called for in the recipes with any you happen to have handy in the house (with the exception of soy oil; it's too thin). You can also add (or change) any scent by using different flavored extracts or fragrant oils.

Massage Procedures

There are a couple of methods to get the most out of your massage:

Steam First, Massage Later Method

If you have a steam room available to you, by all means take advantage of it.   (If a sauna, only, is accessible, be sure to wet your body before you enter and keep re-applying water during your stay so the dry heat doesn't dehydrate your skin.)

Shower first, to get clean.   Then sit – or lie – in the steam room for ten to fifteen minutes or so to open the pores and purge the body of toxins. Next, rinse under a barely cool shower for a minute and pat your body dry. *Now*, let your masseuse and your oils do the rest.

Don't shower, afterward.   Just slip your silky body into something silky.

Massage First, Steam Later Method

Shower first, as usual.   Mildly steam your body for five minutes or so to open the pores.   Pat your body dry and enjoy your massage.   Go back into the steam room for five or ten minutes and let the gentle water particles surround your body to help the oils penetrate.   Step under a cool shower for just a moment to close the pores and refresh you, then simply pat your soft and sleek body dry.

Recipes for Massage Oils

Deep Penetrating Almond Massage Oil

    3   oz almond oil
1 1/2 tsp liquid lecithin
    1   tbsp almond extract

Warm oil and stir in lecithin.   Beat almond extract into oil mixture.   Cool and pour into plastic bottle.   Shake before using. Refrigerate.

Scented Massage Oil

1   tsp liquid lecithin
2   oz soy oil
1   oz peanut oil
1   tbsp oil of any essence you prefer (musk — only 1 tsp be-
     cause the odor is very strong — or sandalwood is nice for a
     man; perhaps a floral scent for a woman; or citrus for both)

Warm first two oils and lecithin lightly. Add scent and cool. Pour into plastic bottle. Refrigerate.

Lemon-Apricot Massage Oil

3   oz apricot oil
1 1/2 tbsp anhydrous lanolin
1   tsp lecithin
1 1/2 tbsp lemon extract

Melt lanolin over low heat. Warm apricot oil and beat into lanolin. Beat in lecithin and let cool. Beat in extract and put in plastic bottle. Refrigerate.

High Friction Massage Cream

1   tbsp beeswax
1   tbsp spermaceti
2   tbsp anhydrous lanolin
2   oz safflower oil
1/8 tsp borax
1   oz rose water
1/4 tsp oil of bergamot

Melt first three ingredients over *low* heat. Warm the oil. Dissolve the borax in heated rose water. Beat the oil into the wax mixture. As it thickens and cools, beat in rose water. When cream forms and is cool, beat in oil of bergamot and scoop into jar. Refrigerate.

Vitamin A, D, and E Massage Oil with Lecithin
(unscented)

2   oz almond oil
1   oz wheat germ oil
4   vitamin A & D capsules
1 1/2 tsp liquid lecithin

Warm oils and stir in lecithin. When cool, pierce vitamin capsules and empty contents into oil. Put in plastic bottle and shake before using. Refrigerate.

Muscle Massage Oil (for aches and pains)

2   oz anhydrous lanolin
2   oz sesame oil
1   tsp methyl salicylate (oil of wintergreen)
1 1/2 tsp menthol

Melt lanolin over low heat. Warm oil and beat into lanolin. When cool, add methyl salicylate and menthol and put in plastic bottle. DO NOT USE ON FACE and KEEP AWAY FROM CHILDREN.

Favorite Perfume Massage Oil

4   oz safflower oil
2   oz sesame oil
1   tsp lecithin
1   tbsp favorite perfume or cologne

Warm oils slightly and stir in lecithin until completely blended. When mixture is cool, shake in plastic bottle with perfume. Shake before each use and keep in refrigerator when not in use.

Skin Bleaches

Some men and women are plagued with dark spots on (usually) their hands and face. This dark pigment can often be bleached with perseverance and patience. However, even then, the bleach is usually temporary, so don't expect miracles. Bleach creams that you buy in a store are often a compound of ammoniated mercury which is very strong and generally not recommended for continual use.

Ascorbic acid preparations are safer and also have properties which are effective in decreasing the pigment formation as well as helping to remove already fixed pigment.

If one of the following recipes doesn't improve the condition within six or eight weeks, I would advise a visit to the dermatologist. If your doctor finds that they are nothing more serious than "liver spots," and no bleach cream seems to work, you can more often than not cover the spots remarkably well with makeup.

Recipes for Skin Bleaches

Lemon 'n' Glycerin Bleach

1   oz freshly squeezed and strained lemon juice
1   tbsp glycerin

Shake together well in small bottle and apply frequently.

Lemon Bleach Lotion

3   oz fresh, strained lemon juice
1   tbsp alcohol
2   tsp glycerin

Shake together in small bottle and apply frequently.

On-the-Spot Bleach

If you're cooking with lemons, rub the raw lemon over spots before you throw it away. If making a salad, rub lemon and a drop of the oil into spots.

Rose Water Bleach

2   oz rose water
2   oz 17 volume hydrogen perioxide*

Shake together in small bottle and apply frequently.

Glycerin Bleach

1   oz glycerin
1   oz 17 volume hydrogen peroxide*

Shake together in small bottle and apply frequently.

Bleach Cream

2   tsp anhydrous lanolin
2   tsp spermaceti
3   oz petroleum jelly
1   tbsp 17 volume hydrogen peroxide*

Melt first three ingredients together over low heat. Cool. Mix peroxide thoroughly into mixture and put in jar. Apply frequently.

Recipes for Freckle Bleaches

Some people like freckles. Some people don't. If you don't, you might try one of the following:

*Some druggists carry peroxide only in 10 and 20 volume. If you find that to be the case, ask him to mix you up some 17 volume.

Freckle Lotion

3 oz alcohol
1 tsp rose water
1 tbsp tincture of benzoin
1 1/2 tsp benzoic acid
1 oz lemon juice

Shake together in small bottle and apply morning and night.

Freckle Cream

1 oz anhydrous lanolin
1 tbsp 17 volume hydrogen peroxide*
1 tbsp glycerin

Melt lanolin. Warm glycerin and beat into lanolin. Beat peroxide into mixture and apply freely.

Rum Lotion for Freckles

2 oz fresh, strained lemon juice
1 oz light rum
1 tsp glycerin

Shake together in small bottle and apply freely.

Recipes for Chapped Lips

Vitamin E Ointment

1 oz wheat germ oil
1 oz petroleum jelly

---

*Some druggists carry peroxide only in 10 and 20 volume. If you find that to be the case, ask him to mix you up some 17 volume.

Melt jelly over low heat. Warm oil and beat into jelly. Beat until cool and put in small jar. Apply before going out into the weather or under lipstick.

Rose Water and Glycerin Lotion

1   oz rose water
1   oz glycerin

Shake together in bottle and apply freely.

Chapped Lip Butter

1   oz cocoa butter
1   tsp spermaceti
1   tsp almond oil

Melt cocoa butter and spermaceti over low heat. Beat in almond oil and continue beating until cool. Pour into small jar and apply freely.

Chapped Lip Stick

1   tbsp beeswax
1   tbsp spermaceti
1   oz olive oil
1   oz petroleum jelly

Melt waxes over low heat. Warm oil and beat into wax mixture. Beat until cool and scoop into lipstick cases. Recipe fills *two* cases.

Coconut Chapped-Lipstick

1 1/2 tbsp beeswax
   1   tbsp spermaceti
   1   tbsp coconut oil

Melt waxes over low heat. Warm coconut oil and beat into wax mixture until cool. Scoop mixture (it's easiest to use your fingers) into empty, clean lipstick cases and pack down well. Recipe will fill *two* lipstick cases. Use freely as you would lipstick.

Recipes for Nails

Nailpolish Remover

6   oz acetone
4   oz alcohol

Shake together in bottle.

Cuticle Softener

vegetable oil of your choice

That's all. Warm oil and dip fingertips into it for a couple of minutes. Massage oil well into cuticles and fingers. (Or massage into entire hand and wear gloves to bed.) Do this once a week; after manicure but before applying polish is a good time.

Fragrances

Custom Colognes

You can purchase the essential oil of any scent you desire at either the drug or health food store. (Candle stores and department stores usually carry scents as well.) Apply it full strength or dilute it with alcohol or witch hazel to any consistency or strength you like.

Cream Sachet

1   tbsp beeswax
1   tbsp light mineral oil
1-2   tsp essential oil (scent of your choice)

Melt beeswax over low heat. Warm mineral oil slightly and beat into wax. Beat in scented oil until sachet is cool and semisolid. Scoop into small container with air-tight cover. (A small pill jar is perfect. Be sure the opening is large enough for your finger.)

Recipe for Sweet Breath

After eating garlic or onions, chew a little raw parsley.

Recipes for Simple Kitchen Burns

It's a good idea to keep one of these ready and waiting in the refrigerator in case of an emergency. In cases of a burn, flood the area with cold water, pat dry, and apply the soothing or healing ointment of your choice.

Aloe Ointment

1 aloe plant

Keep it growing on the kitchen shelf. That's all. Simply break off a leaf and smear the sap onto the burn. It relieves and heals at the same time.

Vitamin A Oil

cod liver oil

Apply it straight. Just rub it on the burned area. This is an excellent healer for even rather severe burns.

Tea and Soda Burn Relief

Mix enough strong, dark tea with baking soda to form a spreadable paste. Apply locally to burn.

Lime Lotion for Burns

3   oz lime water
3   tbsp vegetable oil
1   tsp borax
1   tsp tincture of benzoin

Shake first three ingredients in bottle. Add tincture of benzoin. Keep in refrigerator for emergency burns.

Hand Lotions

Next to the skin on your face, that on your hands gets the most abuse. Especially if they're subjected to frequent soap and water or detergent dips.

The following creams are ultrarich, moisturizing, and protective, so for repeated daily applications a little is all you need each time.

For more serious treatments, hands luckily respond very well to overnight conditioning. Simply get a pair of inexpensive cotton gloves at the dime store. Just before you turn out the light at night, smother your hands with one of the following creams or lotions, put the gloves on, and let the moisturizers do their wonder-work the whole night through. You'll probably see lovely results the very first morning. (Same procedure can be used for calloused feet – use cotton socks.)

You can give yourself a treatment during the day, too. If you clean house or wash dishes with rubber gloves, rub some vegetable oil into your hands before donning the gloves. The heat and perspiration inside the gloves help the oil penetrate and soften your hands.

Recipes for Hand Creams

Do not substitute oils. These were selected for their lightness. If you substitute, the cream will be too gooey to use on your hands.

Lanolin Hand Cream

4   tbsp anhydrous lanolin
1   tbsp plus 1 tsp safflower oil
1 1/2 tsp rose water
1/2   tsp oil of bergamot

Melt lanolin and beat in warmed safflower oil. Heat rose water and beat into mixture, pouring very slowly, until cool. Beat in oil of bergamot and put in jar. Don't worry if it doesn't seem thick enough; it will thicken further in the jar. Makes about 3 oz.

Glycerin and Rose Water Hand Cream

2   tbsp anhydrous lanolin
1   oz glycerin
1/2   oz light mineral oil
1 1/2 tsp soy oil
1   oz rose water
1   tbsp oil of roses (or other floral oil)

Melt lanolin over low heat. Warm next three ingredients together and beat into lanolin. Heat rose water slightly and beat into mixture until it thickens and cools. Beat in scented oil and put in jar. Makes a little over 3 oz.

Orange Hand Cream

2   tbsp anhydrous lanolin
2   tbsp petroleum jelly
1   tbsp glycerin
1/2   tsp boric acid
1   tbsp orange extract

Melt lanolin and petroleum jelly over low heat. Heat glycerin and boric acid slightly and beat into mixture.

Slightly warm orange extract and beat into mixture until cool. Makes 3 oz.

Lemon Hand Cream

3   oz anhydrous lanolin
1   oz soy oil (do not substitute)
1   tbsp glycerin
1   tbsp cocoa butter
1   tsp zinc oxide ointment
2   tsp lemon oil

   Melt lanolin. Warm soy oil, glycerin, and cocoa butter together and beat into lanolin. Beat in zinc oxide and lemon oil until cool. Makes 4 oz.

Almond Hand Cream

4   oz anhydrous lanolin
2   oz almond oil
2   oz almond extract
2   tbsp glycerin
2   tsp zinc oxide ointment
1   tsp boric acid

   Melt lanolin over low heat. Warm glycerin and oil and beat into lanolin. Dissolve boric acid in almond extract and beat into mixture until cool. Beat in zinc oxide. Makes 4 oz.

Your Favorite Scent Hand and Body Lotion

2   tbsp anhydrous lanolin
3   oz sesame oil
1   tbsp plus 1 tsp favorite extract, perfume or cologne (strongly scented)
1/4 tsp borax

Melt lanolin over low heat.   Warm oil and beat into lanolin.   Dissolve borax in heated extract or perfume and, pouring slowly, beat into mixture.   Beat for at least five minutes until cool and creamy.   Put in dispenser bottle. (This is my favorite for everyday use.   It smells heavenly, penetrates quickly and softens beautifully.)   Makes 5 oz.

Glycerin and Rose Water Hand and Body Lotion

3   oz rose water
3   oz glycerin
1/4   oz borax
2   drops red food coloring

Warm glycerin.   Dissolve borax in heated rose water and beat into glycerin until cool.   Beat in food coloring and put in bottle and shake before each use.   Makes 6 oz.

11

Cleopatra to You

If the nose of Cleopatra had been a little shorter, it would have changed the history of the world.

—Blaise Pascal

Cleopatra is reputed to have originated home cosmetics by applying lampblack to her lashes and discovering the milk bath. But a manuscript dating from 1200 B.C., long before Cleopatra, listed dozens of recipes for beauty that were to be prepared by Egyptian women those thousands of years ago. It even used some of the same ingredients you'll find in this book. . .such as thyme, fresh fruits, and sesame oil. So Cleopatra, in the forties and fifties B.C., wasn't the first home cosmetician. And I, in the (19)70s A.D., wouldn't pretend to be, either.

Researchers in the fields of anthropology, archeology, and ethnology appear to agree, however, that the use of cosmetics *did* originate in Egypt. But in Egypt B.C. (before Cleopatra). The earliest records reveal that they were employed in conjunction with religious ceremonies.

King Tutankhamen's 3 1/2 thousand year old tomb, when opened in the 1920s revealed a large number of jars *still* containing cosmetics. (!) When analyzed, they were found to be made primarily of animal fats (which you won't find used extensively in this book.)

Evidence also suggests that other ancient cultures, such as China and India, maintained comparable religious practices, complete with the use of cosmetics. It is known, for example, that the ancient Hindus made great use of almond paste (which you will find recommended in this book).

One might think of Egypt and its counterpart cultures as kind of the "Ceremonial Cosmetic Era." Whenever a woman living in the ancient world anointed her body, she could always say it was for "religious purposes."

The high priests of those religions, however, had a better idea for cosmetics and took the beauty account with them when they slipped over from religion to medicine — if "medicine" it could be called. The art of healing ("science" was unknown) was still sprinkled liberally with astrology, magic, and mysticism.

In their new practice of medicine the priests used cosmetics to ward off physical devils whereas in their former professions they had used them to ward off spiritual ones. The Egyptian ladies didn't seem to care which devils the beauty aids were supposed to "ward off" as long as it wasn't the mortal ones. And so for the next few thousand years they could pretend they were applying mud masks for "medicinal purposes."

There was even a grain of truth in that one, but medicine, itself, was inextricably bound to religion and a long way from assuming its proper place as a science.

It wasn't until around the fifth century B.C. in Greece (which *still* antedates Cleopatra) that medicine was separated from medicine men and mysticism. Hippocrates advanced skin care in particular when he formulated the study of dermatology. He also advocated proper diet, exercise, baths, and massages as aids toward physical health and beauty.

Cosmetology, as such, was of course not yet dreamed of as a separate study, but soon, medical schools were established in many Greek states, and beauty aids were in popular use as they took their place within the larger concept of human health.

New values were born with the Greeks. Among them were the values of ideas, of *scientific* exploration, of man's body, of man's mind. . . of Man. The Greeks' adoration of the heroic in Man led them logically, not mystically, to promote the health and adornment of man himself. People, for the first time, did not have to pretend they were using cosmetics to appease a demon god or to scare off a monstrous plague or pox. An entire culture recognized the use of them as a rational aid toward human health and its resulting beauty. . .for its own sake.

The ideas and practices of the Greeks (including those relating to cosmetics and beauty) were to form the cornerstone for all of future civilization. And their innovations would be preserved and disseminated by two major groups until the Renaissance. The scholars would preserve them. And the armies would disseminate them.

We are, of course, indebted to the Greek scholars first for *originating* and transcribing Greek thought. Aristotle (384-322 B.C.) was unquestionably the greatest. Aside from his unprecedented achievements in other subjects — most notably philosophy — he advanced the cause of beauty as well by offering totally new concepts in biology and physical science. He also systemized the study of botany.

Erasistratos (258 B.C.) propelled cosmetics another leap forward when he established physiology as a separate study and delineated the separate functions of hygienic and therapeutic care of the body.

It was Aristotle's teachings that were to have unending influence, however. Since he was the private tutor of Alexander the Great, his ideas were transported personally to other lands — Persia, India, and Egypt — as Alexander and his armies conquered the world.

Later, the Romans rejected the philosophical bases of Greek thought — they were particularly reluctant to consider "foreign" ideas on medicine and health at first — but they eagerly adopted the arts resulting from them. And the art of personal embellishment soared to dizzying heights prompted by their bacchanalian lifestyle.

In the first century A.D., Crito, a Roman writer, published *four* books on the making of cosmetics. One of them alone included recipes for 1) the preservation and increases of the growth of hair, 2) dye for gray hair, 3) bleaching and golden tinting of hair, 4) greasing of hair, 5) avoidance of wrinkles, 6) acquiring a clear skin, 7) eyebrow pencils, 8) care of nails, 9) decrease in mouth odors, 10) perspiration ointments, 11) aromatic odors for the body.

Another more important scholar by the name of Galen crystallized the values of personal beauty and health in his studies on anatomy, physiology, hygiene, pharmacy, and more. He is also credited with the invention of the first cold cream.

Although these, and other scholars, served to amplify many of the constructs of Greek thought, the philosophical atmosphere of the Roman culture as a whole resulted in a concentration on the practical. . .the immediate. Consequently, many Greek customs were merely copied by the Romans without an understanding of *why* the customs had developed. Therefore, while the Romans were in many ways brilliantly inventive in their applications and extensions of those Greek practices, the era was fundamentally one of indulgence, and with Rome ruling the world, beauty and all of its products became the handmaidens of physical pleasure.

The customs of the Greeks were flowing east as well. Not as a result of war, as in the case of Rome, but because of the migration of teachers. When the Academy of Athens, which had been established by Plato, was closed, a handful of the professors became resident in the court of Persia. There they were able to introduce afresh their ideas on philosophy, science, and medicine.

Persia, along with Syria, Judea, Mesopotamia, Egypt, and Spain, would soon be conquered by the rising power of the Muslins. And with the fall of Rome in 476 A.D., the spotlight of influence soon shifted to the Islamic peoples — mostly Arab.

Customs shifted, too — and with no particular consistency in kind. The Arabs tried to improve themselves by taking what they thought was the best from each culture they ruled. And because the caliphs conscientiously ordered foreign works translated into Arabic; Hippocrates, Aristotle, and Galen formed a stable triad of knowledge upon which was built the rational frame of the Muslim culture.

However, because, like Rome, the Arabs adopted the *practices* rather than the *principles* of Greece, their era was fundamentally one of *assimilation* rather than *advancement*, and the status of beauty was affected accordingly.

The light of Rome had already been extinguished and when the Arab influence waned as well, the world and most of its beauty on all levels was plunged into total darkness for hundreds of years.

The "Middle Ages" have been called "a thousand years without a bath." And it nearly was. Disease was rampant, and skin conditons were not exempt. But because people suffering from any such condition were considered to be unclean, monks (the most learned men of the time) were not allowed, by law, to treat them. The job fell to anyone who would accept it. . .whether or not he was qualified. More often than not, the local barber attended to skin ailments.

During this shriveled feudal era, the hope of civilization lay within the hands of a very few guardians who valued knowledge and learning. Once again, the ideas of previous, enlightened civilizations would be painstakingly copied by the academicians — now the monks — who would turn their monasteries into repositories for ancient manuscripts. Beauty, along with most of the rest of life's affirmative concepts, was hopefully preserved and safe-guarded in the frozen form of books.

The light of civilization flickered hesitatingly with Charlemagne who tried to stimulate a desire for learning. And with Alfred the Great who encouraged a return to letters. And with the other few rulers who sent translators to Spain (the greatest legacy of Arab rule) to bring back the works of scientists and physicians which were available in Latin.

But it wasn't until the twelfth century that the flame would catch and promise to survive. Intellectual ambition was recognized as a value again, and scientific ambition in particular was largely headquartered at the university at Salerno in southern Italy. For three hundred years the Christian school, devoted to medicine and science, had struggled to preserve and translate the great works of the ancient scholars.

By 1200 A.D. they had succeeded sufficiently to attract scholars from all over Western Europe who could then stimulate intellectual curiosity in thier own homelands upon their return.

The university was also the first hospital for returning soldiers from the Crusades. Because of this, many English, French, and German soldiers who were treated there would be able to take healthful living habits back to their own native lands.

Creative thinking was germinating in the Mediterranean again. Universities began to spring up (or wake up) all over Western Europe, encouraged by the activity at Saler-no. The ideas that had given birth to Ancient Greece would now give rebirth. . .to the Renaissance.

"Renaissance" *means* "rebirth." Of ideas. Of the *value* of ideas. . .and since man is the only creature who can hold ideas, of the value of *Man*. Soon the arts would not only flourish but *progress* as they had not since the glory of Greece. Other cultures had adopted many of the trappings of Greek thought, but the Renaissance culture grasped many of the *principles* upon which the customs had been based and consequently progressed.

Mind and body were to a large extent reunited, and glorification of the entire phenomenon which was *Man* would become the predominant hallmark of the era. . . in art. . .and in life.

During the Renaissance, great advancement in the cosmetic world was realized. One giant step forward was made in France. The university at Montpellier had accumulated many scholars from Salerno, and so it became a major seat for medical learning.

Henri de Mondeville studied at Montpellier and was to effectively alter if not revolutionize the stature of cosmetics. He wrote a comprehensive textbook primarily on surgery. In it he distinguished most sharply between *medical* treatment for *pathological abnormalities* of the skin and *cosmetic* treatment for the embellishment of *normal* skin. Although the treatise emphasized medical aspects of skin care, he seemed to recognize the desirability of cosmetic products for cosmetic purposes, because in the same book he offered recipes for pomades, ointments, soaps, etc., "to repair the irreparable outrage of years."

The prevailing wind of rationality that directed the course of the Renaissance was to engender another, this time unparalleled, phenomenon which would affect beauty and *women* for the rest of time.

Up until this period, as we have seen, the preservation and dissemination of knowledge was confined largely to the academies and their teachers and/or rulers and their armies. In either case, they were carried out almost exclusively by *men*. The climate of the Renaissance drastically altered the balance of influence between the sexes. That is to say, *women*, for the first time since Cleopatra, had a real voice. Needless to say, this affected the realm of beauty and cosmetics enormously. Because the women who would help mold its future were not physicians, cosmetics would further split from medicine and gain an identity of its own.

The powerful role of women emerged because nations who had heretofore sought out other countries to conquer and plunder by force were now attempting to *avoid* warring with each other. They were learning to *trade*. And they found that they could form friendly alliances by trading, among other things, women of royal birth. Well-planned, royal marriages afforded them blood ties with the rulers of other countries and spared the blood of their own. Dreadful as it may sound to us today (as dreadful it *was*!), when examined within the context of women during that period, it was the beginning of women's emancipation.

Catherine de'Medici, daughter of Lorenzo (one of the most influential leaders of the Renaissance in Florence) was the first young lady of importance to our subject to be "married off." She was an intelligent child who became a shrewd woman; and she was thoroughly skilled in the art of cosmetics.

Travel and royal marriages between different countries began to spread *all* customs at an accelerated pace. Beauty was no exception. When Mary Queen of Scots became the bride of Francois I, she became the daughter-in-law of Catherine de'Medici at the same time. She learned the beauty secrets of the Queen Dowager and, upon the death of Francois, took them with her when she returned to the land of her birth. Scotland and England were impressed.

Mary's cousin, Queen Elizabeth I, became an ardent experimenter with beauty concoctions. She is said to have invented a perfume. The recipe, in the event you would like to try it, is as follows: "Take eight spoonfuls of compound water, the weight of twopence in fine sugar and boil it on hot embers and coals softly, (add) the weight of twopence of the powder of benjamin. The perfume is very sweet and good for the time."

Because of such royal interest, cosmetics was beginning to come into its own. Since ancient times, man, and especially his women, had ever been concerned with the use of them. From Egypt to Greece to Rome – with a little detour to Arabia – to Florence to France to England. For the protection of man's body and soul to the glorification of them. And America, who would address herself to the freedom of man – and as a side effect turn the beauty business into a multibillion dollar industry – was not yet even born.

Once France gave cosmetics an identity of its own by finally separating therapeutic and beautifying practices, and the royal ladies and their ladies in turn set the fashion, women all over Europe had a heyday. Especially in Protestant England where religious restrictions were more relaxed than on the Continent.

Beauties in Shakespeare's England took the subject so seriously that writers of the day aimed the arrows of their wit at the ladies' preoccupations. From *Love's Labour's Lost:* "Your mistresses dare never come in the rain/For fear their colours should be washed away." Samuel "Hudibras" Butler penned: "Not more than ten among a thousand weare/ Their own complexions or their haire/ That, like their watches, weare their faces/In delicate Inammeld cases."

Up until and through the Victorian age – in spite of Queen Victoria's attempts at restraint – preparing beauty aids at home was approached with such zeal that not only books but magazines as well were published offering recipes.

Women were instructed to use horseradish and cold milk for making a cosmetic to improve the hue and condition of the skin.   Those who were too shy to buy the ingredients for making rouge from the chemist were urged to rub their cheeks with a piece of bright crimson silk dipped in the spirit of wine.   And coconut oil was recommended to lengthen eyelashes.

With all of this wholesale indulgence in the use of cosmetics, it seems inconceivable that women were still making their concoctions *at home.*   The first *pharmacopoeia of London* as early as 1618(!) showed that pharmacists had the equipment and know-how to make and sell cosmetics; and it's quite clear that the demand was there. What, then, prevented that next logical step of selling cosmetics ready-made?

The government stopped it even before it was started by placing such stringent regulations upon the trade that pharmacologists were forced to restrict their talents to the compounding of medicines alone.   They were allowed to sell only the separate ingredients for cosmetics.   The progress of cosmetics was blocked again.

It had taken a few thousand years for medicine to flourish because it was shackled by religion.   Then it took another couple of thousand years for the science of *cosmetics* to emerge because *it* was shackled by medicine. Now, the cosmetic *industry* was strangled before it was even born because it was shackled by *government.*

America would give it birth.

The American Indians had already influenced the cosmetic practices of Europe.   By using natural fats as a base for ceremonial paints, they protected their skin and were able to more easily remove the paint.   Sixteenth-century English explorers took this information back home with them, and women all over Europe began using under-makeup moisturizers for the first time.

Many of the first settlers in America were poor.   Many of them were rough.   Many had religious convictions demanding simple adornment and dress.   None of them knew much about the art of beautification. The ones who might have been interested had not even been familiar with cosmetics in the countries of their birth because they hadn't been able to afford the ingredients, so no one could say the cosmetic industry in America flourished immediately.

Some of the women evidently knew enough to tie a bit of bacon to their faces before bed (protein, but can you imagine???), but it wasn't until the arrival of the aristocracy in the eighteenth century that cosmetics became familiar items and began to be at all popular in the colonies. And even then they were used to a limited degree. Americans were forced to purchase scents, powders, and the essential "fixings" for beauty aids from England, and because of the heavy taxation the cost was prohibitive to most colonists.

A few women, mostly widows who needed a means of supporting themselves, went into business, advertised and sold their homemade creams and beauty aids. But because of the previously mentioned difficulty in obtaining the ingredients and some of the same strict regulations by the very government that was stifling English business, they failed to reach any degree of success.

Another problem for the colonists was that even the bottles and jars to *hold* the cosmetics had to come from England. That problem was relieved somewhat in 1763 when the first glass house was opened in Pennsylvania.

By that time, however, nobody was much interested in pursuing beauty. Americans had become single-minded in their interest of pursuing freedom.

From the Revolution until James Madison became President of the United States, beauty and cosmetics played an unimportant role — if any role at all — in the culture.

It was President Madison's wife, Dolley, who brought beauty, glamour, and cosmetics back to the attention of

American women. And her influence predominated only in the South. The North was still depriving itself of many pleasures, including beautifying cosmetics, under the cold eye of the Puritans.

But the seeds of energy had been sown with the achievement of freedom, and no one, including the Puritans, could nip the blooming of America.

The nineteenth century was a century of progress built upon progress. America was scrambling to her feet economically as the system of free enterprise rocketed her from one astounding advancement to another. Relieved of the yokes of religious oppression, tyrannical rulers, and, to a large extent, government intervention, men created and produced at an accelerated rate.

Just to mention a couple of stepping stones in the progress of beauty products, Theron T. Pond in 1846 offered "Pond's Extract" to the public. And in 1847, Salon Palmer started his own line of cosmetics. . .including powders, colognes, and lotions. He was the first person in the world to distribute a complete line of cosmetics under one name.

The imaginations of two other Americans, in particular, influenced cosmetics by paving the way for *mass production* and *mass marketing.* V. Chapin Dagget came up with the idea of substituting white mineral oil for the perishable vegetable oils which had been used previously in the making of creams. Unlimited shelf life for creams was possible because of this. Next, Henry Tetlow found that zinc oxide made a good, *cheap* base for face powder which resulted in rouges and powders becoming accessible to women who could never have afforded "store bought" cosmetics before. Because businessmen could enter the market with so little capital, many of them began to get into the cosmetic field by selling powders. A number of large cosmetic houses existing today got their start with a few boxes of powder.

And so *we* arrive. . .women of the twentieth century. We find ourselves surrounded by a far greater number and variety of beauty concoctions than were prepared by all of our historical sisters combined.

The fact is that *only* a woman in such a setting of plenty would find the idea of a book devoted to the making of her own beauty aids a novel one. As we have seen, *ready-made* cosmetics were available for the first time – and then in very limited number and kind – in the nineteenth century. And it wasn't until technology gained momentum in the twentieth century that the industry started its rush up to today's staggering heights. We take ready-made cosmetics for granted to such a degree that it is shocking to realize that it wasn't until as late as 1951 that the beauty industry in the United States hit one billion dollars for the first time. And today, barely twenty-five years later, the market is veritably flooded with a mind-boggling selection of beauty aids on which American women (and men) spend ten billion dollars a year.

Two unique phenomena separate and distinguish us from the ladies of history. One is modern woman herself, and her mentality. It's high. She asks the question, "Why?" "Why is this product beneficial to my skin?" "What's in it that makes it so good?" And that's *why* making cosmetics at home is such a good thing. After you understand what your skin is all about – what its nature is, and what its requirements are for health and beauty – then you can custom create cosmetics by combining the exact ingredients that fulfill your own *individual* needs.

The second distinguishing characteristic is the time and place in which we find ourselves. We are *free to ask* the question "Why?" And we have the child of that freedom – technology. It just so happens that Cleopatra had a pretty good idea when she soaked in her milk bath. But can you conceive of the *amount of time* and the *number of slaves* required to milk by *hand* how many(?) animals to get *enough milk to fill a bathtub?*

All *we* have to do is open a packet of powdered milk and run it under the tap. What we sometimes forget is that packets of milk don't "grow" in the supermarket.

An animal was nourished by the latest scientific methods and milked by machine. The milk was kept sterile and fresh in containers manufactured by a company employing many people employing more machines. The containers protecting the milk were carried by trucks on super highways and trains on super steel at speeds of up to and over one hundred miles an hour to another factory. There the milk was dried by a process a man invented exactly for that purpose and put into packages which were manufactured by another company, who bought the paper from another, which was printed by yet another. Modern woman buys it at the grocery store for ten cents a pack, pours the contents into her bathtub, turns a faucet, and within five minutes is sinking into a bath as rich, with equally as much softening and whitening power, as Cleopatra ever expected from hers.

Cosmetics are free at last. Once mass production was made possible, knowledge grew at a furious pace. The cosmetics industry employs both doctors and scientists to extend the concepts of cosmetic products and possibilities. They also, through advertising, educated the American woman on a mass level as they forged ahead with new ideas. Ironically, it's because of the progress and communication of the cosmetic industry that modern woman no longer needs to buy her beauty aids. Cosmetics are now liberated even from the standardization of mass-produced goods.

And many of us do want more than those mass-produced products can offer. We want more than a middle-of-the-road beauty aid which is only "generally" right for our individual skin type, requirements, and tastes. We want products *exactly* and specifically designed and created for each of us. And the only way to get a custom-made product like that is to custom make it.

So we can blithely brew away with our blenders, juicers, and mixers, adopt and adapt new ideas offered by the cosmetics industry, and create our very own products at home.

But *we* have a choice. We can purchase or produce. Our counterparts in history might say that we have the best of both worlds. Theirs and ours.

For there's nothing mystical in our world of beauty. Your religion, if you have one, won't affect the condition of your skin. And putting yogurt on your face may scare away a caller or two, but not any evil spirits.

Modern-day *beauty* is the crisp, no-nonsense intelligence of modern-day *woman* put into action. . .with, of course, a little help from Mother Nature's gifts, man's technology and knowledge, fifteen minutes in a modern kitchen, *and* a copy of this book.

12

The Beauty
Gourmet's Glossary

INGREDIENT	DEFINITION	WHERE TO BUY
Acetone	A colorless, volatile, water-soluble, flammable liquid. Used in nailpolish removers.	Drugstore
Alcohol	Reducing agent. Cools skin as evaporates; reduces perspiration. Antiseptic with drying power. Skin cleanser to remove skin debris.	Drugstore
Almonds	A nutlike kernel; fruit of the almond tree. Source of protein with abrasive action.	
Almond oil	Emollient. Natural vegetable oil pressed from almonds. Held to have most penetrating and softening power.	Health food store or super- market
Aloe	Any chiefly African, liliaceous plant of the genus Aloe, certain species of which yield a drug and a fiber. Sap used to relieve and heal burns.	Plant store
Alum	A colorless, odorless, crystalline, water-soluble solid. Mild astringent. Mild germicide.	Drugstore

INGREDIENT	DEFINITION	WHERE TO BUY
Apples	Fruit whose juice contains mild organic acids, pectins, protein, and vitamins.	Supermarket
Baking soda	A white crystalline, water-soluble powder or granules. Antacid, reduces greasiness of skin, removes crusts and secretions. Used to soothe burns.	Supermarket
Barley	A cereal plant whose awned flowers grow in tightly bunched spikes. Thought to have properties to cleanse and soften the skin.	Supermarket
Beeswax	Substance secreted on underside of the bee which it uses to build up walls and cells of honeycomb. Will not clog pores and tends to soften skin.	Drugstore*
Benzoic acid	A white, crystalline, slightly water-soluble powder usually derived from benzoin or other balsams.	Drugstore
Bergamot (oil of)	Begamot is a small citrus tree having fruit whose rind yields a fragrant essential oil. Used in small quantities to perfume creams. Also has tanning properties.	Drugstore
Borax	A white, water-soluble powder or crystals occurring naturally or obtained from naturally occurring borates. Used as an emulsifying agent to make blending less difficult.	Drugstore
Boric acid	Antiseptic, fungicide, mild germicide.	Drugstore
Bran	The partly ground husk of wheat or other grain, separated from flour meal by bolting. Thought to act as a skin softener.	Supermarket

*(If you cannot find, you may order direct from Theodor Leonhard Wax Co., 136 Church St., Haledon, N.J. 07508. Price approx. $2.50 per pound + postage — enough for you and all your friends for a year!)

INGREDIENT	DEFINITION	WHERE TO BUY
Brandy	A spirit distilled from the fermented juice of grapes or other fruit. Has modified attributes of alcohol.	Liquor store
Brewer's yeast	A yeast suitable for use as a ferment in the manufacture of wine and beer. Source of much vitamin B.	Health food store or super- market
Calamine powder	A pink, water-insoluble powder consist- ing of zinc oxide and about 0.5% fer- ric oxide, used in ointments, lotions, and the like. Mild astringent, protec- tive dehydrant.	Drugstore
Camphor	A whitish, translucent, crystalline, pleasant-odored antiseptic obtained from the camphor tree. Counter- irritant, its action depends upon be- numbing influence upon peripheral sensory nerves. Gives sense of coolness.	Drugstore
Carrots	Vegetable. Source of vitamin A used to unplug pores and facilitate oil release.	
Castile soap	A variety of mild soap, made from olive oil.	Drugstore
Castor oil	A colorless to pale yellow viscid liquid, usually obtained from the castor bean by pressing process. Emol- lient, lubricant adherent.	Drugstore
Chamomile	Plant having strongly scented foliage and flowers which are used medicinal- ly. Having characteristics of soothing the skin and slight bleaching powers.	Super- market
Cinnamon (oil of)	Germicide, astringent; antiseptic spice oil.	Drugstore
Cocoa butter	A fatty substance obtained from the seeds of the cacao, a small evergreen tree. Emollient and vehicle as well as lubricant for skin's surface.	Drugstore

INGREDIENT	DEFINITION	WHERE TO BUY
Coconut oil	Emollient oil, lubricant, and vehicle pressed from coconuts.	Health food store or super-market
Cornstarch	Starch made from Indian corn. Source of protein with slight abrasive action.	
Cottonseed oil	Emollient, vehicle, lubricant. Natural vegetable oil.	Health food store or super-market
Cucumbers	Vegetable whose juice contains organic acids. Astringent.	Super-market
Epsom salts	Hydrated magnesium sulfate occurring as small colorless crystals. Supposed to exercise osmotic influence on inflammatory tissue. Has slight anesthetic effect.	Drugstore
Extracts	Preparations supposed to possess the virtue of the original substance in concentrated form.	Super-market
Fuller's earth	An absorbent clay, used especially for removing grease from fabrics. Absorbent face mask ingredient.	Drugstore
Gelatin	Adhesive yet porous dressing. Protective, supportive, permits evaporation of secretions through it. Protein.	Super-market
Gin	An alcoholic liquor obtained by distilling grain mash with juniper berries. Same antiseptic qualities as alcohol.	Liquor store
Glycerin	Clear, sweet, odorless substance. By-product of oils and fats. Mild antiseptic, emollient when dilute. Absorbent, hence used to prevent drying of many preparations. Facilitates penetration through epidermis according to some.	Drugstore

INGREDIENT	DEFINITION	WHERE TO BUY
Honey	A sweet, viscid fluid produced by bees from the nectar collected from flowers. When applied to skin, has remarkable drawing power plus moisturizing qualities.	Health food store or super-market
Hydrogen peroxide	A colorless, unstable oily liquid, H_2O_2, the aqueous solution of which is used chiefly as an antiseptic and bleaching agent.	Drugstore
Hydro-genated oils	Oils which through treatment become hardened. Margarine and lard substitute.	Super-market
Iodine	A nonmetallic halogen element. Used in preparations as an antiseptic coloring agent.	Drugstore
Lanolin	Purified fat from sheep wool. Pro-tective ointment base which combats dryness and softens locally on the surface; it is said to contain elements similar to those of our own sebaceous glands and so is readily absorbed by the skin.	Drugstore
Lecithin	Any of a group of yellow-brown fatty substances occurring in animal and plant tissues and egg yolk. Emul-sifying agent; lowers surface tension between oils and water, hence aiding absorption through skin.	Health food store or super-market
Lemon	Citrus fruit used as a skin freshener and bleach. Astringent.	Super-market
Lime water	Antacid, astringent, antiseptic; used for burns.	Drugstore
Margarine	A food product made from a blend of refined vegetable oils churned with ripened skim milk, with a plastic consistency. Penetrating skin lubricant.	Super-market

INGREDIENT	DEFINITION	WHERE TO BUY
Menthol	A colorless, crystalline, slightly water-soluble alcohol obtained from peppermint oil. Local sedative, antiseptic, counterirritant.	Drugstore
Methyl salicylate (oil of wintergreen)	Perfume, antiseptic. Penetrating qualities helpful to aches and pains. Poison.	Drugstore
Mineral oils	Cheaper oils usually used in cosmetics. Is nonabsorbent. Can cleanse surface and lubricate.	Drugstore
Mineral water	Water containing dissolved mineral salts or gases, especially such water for medicinal use.	Super-market
Oatmeal	Protein meal made from oats. Used for its abrasive qualities.	Super-market
Olive oil	Natural oil pressed from olives. Emollient, lubricant with excellent penetrating powers.	Health food store or super-market
Orange water	Neutral reaction to slightly acid. Light orange odor.	Health food store or drug-store
Papaya	The large, yellow, melonlike fruit of a tropical shrub or small tree. Exfoliant containing active enzymes which are capable of eating up dead skin cells on the surface of the skin.	Super-market
Peach kernel oil	Natural vegetable oil. Can substitute for almond or olive oil.	Health food store or super-market

INGREDIENT	DEFINITION	WHERE TO BUY
Peanut oil	Natural vegetable oil from peanuts. Can substitute for almond or olive oil.	Health food store or supermarket
Peppermint	A labiate herb known for its refreshing and drawing qualities. Antiseptic.	Supermarket
Petroleum jelly	A yellowish or whitish, translucent, gelatinous, oily semisolid. Nonpenetrable lubricant; protective base.	Drugstore or supersupermarket
Phenol	Antiseptic; germicide.	Drugstore
Rosemary	An evergreen native to the Mediterranean area. Herb used in medicines and cosmetics.	Supermarket
Rose water	Water tinctured with the essential oil of roses. Wholly free of irritants.	Drugstore
Sage	A perennial herb used in medicines, cookery, and believed to have a drying effect upon the skin.	Supermarket
Salt	A crystalline compound occurring as a mineral, a constituent of sea water. Antiseptic, abrasive.	Health food store or supermarket
Sesame oil	Natural oil pressed from sesame seeds. Promotes skin softeness and absorbs high percentage of sun's ultraviolet rays.	Health food store or supermarket
Skim milk	Milk from which most of the fat has been removed. Protein, skin softener, mild bleach.	Supermarket
Sodium benzoate	A white, crystalline or granular water-soluble powder. Antiseptic; natural perservative.	Drugstore

INGREDIENT	DEFINITION	WHERE TO BUY
Soybean oil	Natural vegetable oil pressed from soybeans.	Health food store or super-market
Spermaceti	Emollient, demulcent, hardening ingredient from the head of a whale. Softens skin and will not clog pores.	Drugstore
Straw-berries	Fruit whose juice contains organic acids. Astringent. Thought to have exceptional skin cleansing qualities.	Super-market
Tannic acid	Characteristic of tea that soothes skin, especially burns.	Super-market
Thyme	A common garden herb having aromatic leaves. Attributes of antiseptic and disinfectant.	Drugstore
Thymol	Antiseptic similar to phenol.	Drugstore
Tincture of benzoin	Adds sticking quality, protective antiseptic; astringent; irritant. Used to aid the healing of erupted skins.	Drugstore
Tragacanth	Substance derived from low, spiny Asian shrubs. Demulcent, emulsifying agent.	Drugstore
Vodka	An unaged, colorless, distilled spirit, originally made in Russia. Contains characteristics of alcohol.	Liquor store
Witch hazel	A shrub of Eastern North America. Astringent, antiseptic, soothing liquid.	Drugstore
Zinc oxide	Mild astringent, mild skin bleach, adhesive dehyrant. Nontoxic, protective.	Drugstore

LIST OF MEASUREMENTS

1 teaspoon	1/3 tablespoon
1 tablespoon	3 teaspoons
2 tablespoons	1/8 cup (1 ounce)
4 tablespoons	1/4 cup
5 1/3 tablespoons	1/3 cup
8 tablespoons	1/2 cup
16 tablespoons	1 cup
1 cup	1/2 pint
2 cups	1 pint
2 pints	1 quart
4 quarts	1 gallon
1 pound	16 ounces
1 fluid ounce	2 tablespoons
16 fluid ounces	1 pint
1 shot glass	1 fluid ounce (2 tablespoons) (*check your shot glass*; some of them contain 1 1/2 ounces)
a pinch	less than 1/8 teaspoon